THROUGH THE
GLASS WALL

THROUGH THE GLASS WALL

Journeys into the

Closed-Off Worlds of the Autistic

HOWARD BUTEN, PH.D.

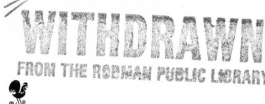

BANTAM BOOKS

THROUGH THE GLASS WALL
A Bantam Book / February 2004

Published by
Bantam Dell
a division of
Random House, Inc.
New York, New York

Book design by Glen Edelstein

Library of Congress Cataloging in Publication Data

Buten, Howard.
    Through the glass wall : journeys into the closed-off
    worlds of the autistic / Howard Buten.
        p. cm.
    ISBN 0-553-80346-8
    1. Autism. 2. Autism—Anecdotes. I. Title.

RC553.A88B88 2004
616.85'882—dc22

                                        2003060686

Manufactured in the United States of America
Published simultaneously in Canada

BVG   10   9   8   7   6   5   4   3   2   1

CONTENTS

Introduction   *1*

1. Hurricanes and Land Mines   3
2. "What Big Eyes You Have!"
    "The Better to Hear You With,
      My Dear!"   51
3. Apples and Oranges   83
4. Imposters   111
5. Playing the Therapeutic Character   143

To Joe Klotz, with gratitude,
and
to the Shelton family, who trusted me

THROUGH THE GLASS WALL

INTRODUCTION

Much has been written about autism. I believe that this has to do with its mystery and its contradictions. The more we know about the little we've learned, the more mysterious and contradictory autism seems to become. Most sentences that begin "Autistic people are . . ." will be necessarily false—there will always be some who aren't.

I began working with these astonishing people back in 1974. Nine years later I felt the need to write about them. I'm a writer; I write. I rewrote the first sentence for a year, trying to make it true, then gave up.

I spent the next twenty years scrupulously not writing the pages that you now hold in your hand. But what I did do during those years was ask myself why it was that I feel—have felt from the very beginning—so at home among the autistic. (*Home:* Where the heart is.) Many colleagues have asked me the same question. When I got tired of not being able to answer them, I decided to write the pages you now hold in your hand. I hoped they might provide me with a few answers. They have.

Here is what this book is not:

It is not a how-to book.

It is not a survey.

It is not a scientific dissertation (though it is often scientific).

It is neither an elegy to the beauty nor a tirade against the horrors of autism.

It is not specifically written for parents of autistic children, whose travails I know intimately but can never truly share, though it may be of interest to them.

It may well be of interest to autism professionals, whose travails, and joys, I do share.

It is not expressly meant to help anyone.

It isn't meant to be a memoir—it's too didactic—but it might be too personal not to be one.

Howard Buten, Ph.D.

1

HURRICANES AND LAND MINES

I work with the autistic, in France. I founded an institution there, a day clinic dedicated to the treatment of extreme cases. I have always been most interested in extreme cases.

When I was a child I wanted to be a doctor—I didn't want to *become* a doctor; I wanted to *be* a doctor, now! I'd found a copy of *Morris's Anatomy* in my cousin Bettie's attic when I was eight years old. I read the whole thing. There were lots of pictures. I memorized the appendectomy procedure—incision, artery, hemostat, suction, section, suture. I felt like a doctor.

At the time I also felt like a ventriloquist; my mother had been a vaudeville performer in her youth, and she'd taught me to sing and dance, so ventriloquism seemed to be the natural next step. I taught myself the basics of the art with the help of a book entitled *So You Want to Be a Ventriloquist?* which I'd come across in the elementary school library while searching for a book that didn't exist but which would have been entitled, had it existed, *So You Want to Be a Brain Surgeon?* Inspired by these two parallel studies, I took to performing two or three appendectomies a week on my ventriloquist dummy (his appendix was a shoelace, inserted in his abdomen the night before, frequently inflamed). A year later my success, as well as that of Christiaan Barnard, allowed me to move on to open-heart surgery (a knotted maroon sock). Both my careers unfortunately came to an abrupt halt with the untimely demise of my dummy, who died of postoperative complications (falling apart at the seams) a few weeks before my tenth birthday.

By the time I was twelve, I was already pursuing three "careers" at the same time: scientist, novelist and performing artist. I wrote my first novel at age twelve, and continued writing a new one every few years. Two years after the tragic death of my ventriloquist dummy, I as scientist won first prize at the Detroit Science Fair for my life-size papier-mâché "Visible Man." As a stage performer, I sang, I danced and I mimed; studied the violin (no talent), the trumpet (almost no talent), then the drums (talent). And by the time I was fourteen, I was spending the first half of my summer vacations as a volunteer in the pathology lab of a large teaching hospital in Detroit where my father knew somebody, cataloguing paraffin samples, carrying test tubes, looking into microscopes. Best of all, I got to wear a white coat, like Dr. Kildare. The second half of my summer vacations, I worked as a volunteer at various camps for various kinds of special children. I spent the first summer as a counselor's aide at the Michigan Muscular Dystrophy Camp. It was here that I perfected my peerless wheelchair-pushing technique: the continuous pushing down and pulling up on the handles from behind, the eye always on the next five yards, anticipating nooks and crannies and hills and dales—a human suspension system ever ready to ensure a smooth ride wherever your destination might take you.

Over the years I worked with inner-city kids, underprivileged psychotic kids, "mongoloid" and retarded kids, inner-city underprivileged mongoloid psychotic kids. I learned the primal lesson of the ineffably narcissistic: doing good for others makes *us* feel good, the ultimate ego trip. One day, suffering from a broken heart and needing to feel good about myself, I took out the Yellow Pages and looked under R, for "Retarded." I thought I'd brush up on Down syndrome—kids so special that they're hardwired for kindness. I was referred to "Special Schools," and there I came across an address not far away. I called. I was given an appointment. I went. What I saw when I got there is why I'm writing this book.

* * *

5

It is 1974. I am twenty-four years old. I am sitting alone in the waiting room of the Children's Orthogenic Center in Detroit, wondering what "orthogenic" means. Suddenly the room is deluged by a hurricane. The hurricane comes in the form of a boy, bursting through the door, throwing himself to the floor, sitting up suddenly, legs out straight and back stiff, rocking back and forth, hands in his lap, eyes staring into middle space, his hoarse voice spitting out syllables as if he'd swallowed something, but hadn't. I have never seen anything like this before in my life. It is stunning. I am stunned . . . and somehow delighted. At twenty-four it is already rare to suddenly see something one has never seen before in one's life. My immediate instinct is to fall on the floor and do as he is doing. I want to know what in the world it could possibly feel like to be him.

I didn't know at the time that this was to be the most burning unanswerable question of my life.

"Extreme cases" may be defined in several ways. One might describe an autistic person who is particularly violent, one who bites, scratches, slaps, spits, bludgeons the people around him—caregivers, family members, other patients—and himself. The term might also apply to those autistics whose pathology makes them extremely hard to get through to (by definition, if you're autistic you're hard to get through to): inert, retarded, difficult to motivate, impossible to move. Or it might also refer to a person who has an extreme effect on the family or on the institutional staff: someone who may be neither violent nor inert, but whose behavior is so disturbing, disruptive or obnoxious that the weight of his or her presence pushes us to extremes.

It was an extreme case that initiated me into my profession, that day in 1974.

The hurricane's name was Adam S. He was four years old. I was to learn later that of the twenty-five-odd youngsters of the Children's Orthogenic Center (*orthogenic* may be defined as for the care and education of children with emotional or cognitive disturbances), Adam S. was the most difficult, the most dangerous. He bit. He bit and he head-butted and he pinched and he pounded, himself as well as others. He had no language. He did not come when called. He would not sit still in a chair. He would sit on the floor at length, however, rocking back and forth, tapping his head backward against the wall; I can still see the bald spot where he'd worn the hair away, a small tempest-tossed island of scalp in a turbulent afro sea.

Adam threw fits. Suddenly, for no apparent reason, he would hurl himself to the ground, flailing his arms, churning his legs, hitting his forehead against whatever surface he found himself on, rolling across it, beside

7

himself, a banshee. We would try to subdue him; it usually took three or four of us. Sometimes we put him in
the time-out room; sometimes we'd stand there, impotent, waiting for the storm to pass.

Adam, autistic, was invulnerable to everything, including pain. I once watched him climb a hurricane
fence, slip and fall to the ground five feet below, flat on
his back, then pick himself up and walk off without so
much as a whimper. It eventually dawned on me that the
boy had an extraordinarily high threshold for pain.
(Certain studies in the 1980s were to demonstrate that
some autistic people have elevated levels of substances
called endogenous opiates—*endogenous* means made by
the body itself—that act as natural painkillers; one of
those opiates is beta-endorphin. This finding would also
help to explain these people's self-injurious behavior:
living in a state of perpetual semi-numbness, they could
be driven to self-mutilation in an unconscious effort to
feel themselves.) I reasoned that if it was true that Adam
did not feel pain as you or I do, he would understandably have trouble distinguishing a caress from a scratch,
a friendly slap on the back from a punch in the nose.
This had to be explained to him. But how? Given his
low level of verbal comprehension, what could we do to
make him understand the difference?

An act of aggression inflicted by someone who does
not distinguish violence from tenderness is aggressive
only if the person receiving it experiences it as such. If a

coconut falls on my head but, thanks to the football helmet that I always wear, doesn't hurt me, no aggression or violence exists; the coconut didn't fall on me on purpose, and I experienced nothing unpleasant.

I decided to create a microcosm wherein Adam's violence would simply not be experienced as such, and thus would not exist. During the summer, the Children's Orthogenic Center was closed for classes, but the building stayed open for consultations. We decided on one-hour sessions, three days a week. I chose a small empty office which was rarely used, with one small window and carpeting on the floor. In the beginning I spent most of my time dodging Adam's teeth, fingernails and fists. I learned to do this calmly, through minimal, fluid movements, a kind of *Aikido* invented for the occasion. I showed no signs of panic, stress or unpleasantness. What I couldn't avoid I simply took, stoically, betraying no reaction whatsoever, practicing a sort of self-hypnosis that renders one invulnerable to pain—or, rather, invulnerable to the slightest reaction to pain; enabled, I suppose, by some primitive survival instinct as well as an extremely self-indulgent Zorro complex. This aside, I spent most of my time imitating Adam, mirroring him: rocking when he rocked, flapping my hands when he flapped his hands, screaming and humming when he screamed and hummed. We crossed our eyes at the same time, flung ourselves against the walls as one, bit ourselves on the hand together, banged our heads in sync.

Outside the little room, Adam followed me everywhere, came when I called, did whatever I asked. My colleagues were dumbfounded.

Time marched on.

It is early August. Adam and I are in session. Adam is standing there in the corner of the little room, making his favorite noise, "sih-sih-sih." (This afternoon's program will also include "Ah-um, ah-um, ah-um UM!" as well as the ever popular "Tik-a-tik-a-tik.") I sing along, standing in the opposite corner. I realize again how pleasant it is to make these noises—the way the air catches in your sinus cavity, the little slapping in your throat, the tiny perpetual suffocations that squeeze and release, squeeze and release. It beats speech by a mile. Suddenly my knees give way—I fall to the floor in sitting position, my legs out straight in front of me. I say, "SIT!" Without the slightest hesitation, Adam falls to the floor in like position and says, "SIH!" A miracle! I can't believe my ears. I grab him and hug him, shake him with joy. He smiles wide. This smile is worth a million dollars, and I want to see it grow. I start to tickle him. I say "Tickle-tickle-tickle" and Adam rolls around the floor, laughing. Now I stop, my hands hovering low over his ribs. He looks at me in anticipation, stares, smiling—then . . . "Ticka!" He says it suddenly and I pounce on him, all ten fingers roiling in his ribs. I stop again. His eyes meet mine. "Ticka!" Adam repeats. *(Cue music.)*

In the coming year Adam will acquire a vocabulary of fifteen words, most but not all of which appear through reciprocal imitation, and all of which are reinforced by a particular pleasure attached to the sense of the word said, an answer to a request on his part—"Rye hoss" (*Ride horse;* we had a rocking horse at the school), "Yowt" (*Yogurt,* one of his favorite foods), etc. As his communication skills increase, Adam's violence dwindles.

The question of what autism is—what it looks like and where it comes from—will be discussed many times in the course of this book. We will see again and again how clear definitions and descriptions turn out to be frustratingly elusive; how they differ from author to author, specialist to specialist, country to country, school of thought to school of thought. This is largely because how autism "looks" often differs from one autistic person to another, from one psychological evaluation to another, from one brain scan to another, from one genetic profile to another. In defining autism, *Blakiston's Pocket Medical Dictionary* makes reference to "thinking unduly influenced by fantasy and daydreaming," whereas, on the contrary, many specialists draw attention to the literal, totally unimaginative nature of autistic thought. Temple Grandin, an autistic woman who is herself a specialist on autism, describes her own inability to mentally conceive metaphors: when she hears someone speak of a "golden door to the future" (at a stockholders' meeting, say), she imagines a very real door, perhaps with a knob and a door frame, that's made of gold. No fantasy and daydreaming here.

There are violent, hyperactive autistic people and there are inert and gentle autistic people; verbal ones and nonverbal ones; heartbreakingly retarded ones and astonishingly brilliant ones; graceful ones and clumsy ones; obsessive-compulsive ones and easy-to-please ones; beautiful ones and ugly ones.

The psychiatrist Leo Kanner, who named the condition in 1943, probably had the simplest, most telling point of view. His distinguishing descriptive criterion was the "air of aloneness" that he observed in these children—the quality they had of behaving as if they were absolutely alone when they were not alone: not noticing others, not reacting to others. To me, it is the presence of this invisible wall that most distinguishes autism from other handicaps and pathologies, and the reason for which autism has often been classified as a communication disorder. This distinction having been made, though, I must confess that I have never encountered, even among the most extreme of the extreme cases, a single autistic person with whom I could not communicate at all, a single autistic person whom I did not, in the end, consider to be "good company."

In certain institutions the most difficult patients are the ones most loved. I consider this to be a good sign. When I came to the Children's Orthogenic Center, Adam S. was the uncontested favorite. He bit.

Adam bit often, bit everyone, bit hard, children and adults alike. He was scolded, screamed at, exiled and upbraided. He was isolated in the time-out room. (In those days "timing-out" was the negative reinforcement of choice. It only dawned on us later that since by definition most severely autistic children seek to be alone with themselves, they are only too delighted to be left in a small room with nothing in it but themselves.) Adam bit; nothing worked. It became evident that radical measures had to be brought to bear. These measures were conceived using the principles of "operant conditioning," a concept to be discussed shortly. Our hearts in hand, it was decided that each staff member be furnished with a small plastic bag, to be worn on the belt, inside of which was a small sponge saturated with Tabasco sauce, of which Adam was to receive a dab in the mouth each time he bit someone. It was loathsome to do, heartbreaking to watch—he shrieked in pain, squirmed on the floor, threw himself against the wall, flailed. Three interminable minutes later we'd grab him up in our arms and collectively comfort him. This protocol, which put everyone's ethical and moral fiber to the test, only served to deepen our affection for the boy.

Adam's biting disappeared in a matter of weeks. It never came back.

Today Adam S. is a strapping young man of thirty-one years. He lives in a group home with three other autistic men. He works in a hotel, uniformed, salaried, helping the chambermaids in their work. He is not totally autonomous. He speaks rarely, but he speaks. He has a bank account. He bought himself a color TV. The clinic I founded in Paris is named after him.

During the years before I came to the Children's Orthogenic Center, I played in rock groups and wrote folk songs. In the sixties, as a political statement, I dropped out of the University of Michigan (major: Chinese language, literature and philosophy) to attend the Ringling Brothers and Barnum & Bailey Clown College. I toured with a small tent circus for two years, and then took my solo clown act to the cabaret/coffeehouse stage. It was the following year that I met Adam S. and discovered autism.

One evening in 1976, in between working at the Children's Orthogenic Center during the day and writing my current novel at night, a well-known comedian spotted me performing at a coffeehouse. Thanks to his generosity, and with great misgivings and everyone's blessing, I left the Children's Orthogenic Center to follow my show business muse to Los Angeles, where, immediately on arrival, I presented myself as a volunteer at the Neuropsychiatric Institute at UCLA. The 5-West ward: autistic and psychotic children.

Naturally, I started imitating the clientele. I was promptly reprimanded for doing so. Members of the staff told me that such imitation would only reinforce the autisms of the autistics. "How do you know that?" I asked. In effect, behaviorism, a school of thought in human psychology that revolutionized the profession in the early seventies, stipulates that "what reinforces what" can be ascertained only through direct observation. "Give me one day," I said. They agreed. The effects— improved communicating and relating—were immediately observable, and I was allowed to continue. I stayed at the institute for three years, thereby surviving my performing career and Hollywood.

During my third year in Los Angeles, my first novel was published (first one published, that is; fifth written) and I moved to New York, where I was accepted into the local study cluster of a nationwide Ph.D. program in clinical psychology. The novel was a failure in the United States, but was published in French translation in Paris in 1981 and became a cult best-seller in France. So a year later, in 1982, I was invited to come to the City of Lights for a week of promotion, and while there was introduced to Dr. Tony Lainé, a well-known French psychiatrist who ran a day clinic for autistic children in the southern Parisian suburbs. He offered me an internship at the clinic, and it was perfect timing. My doctoral program required a year's internship, and the fact that I had already managed to fall madly in love with a French woman made the decision easy. I took him up on his offer.

My year's internship lasted two years. I was much appreciated in general, but my particular style of working with the autistic eventually became problematic to the clinic's powers that be. I was sanctioned for my inability to adapt to the institution's theoretical stance, which was based largely on the psychoanalytic writings of Bruno Bettelheim and a recently deceased post-Freudian psychoanalyst named Jacques Lacan. Bettelheim believed that autism was caused, consciously or unconsciously, by unaffectionate parenting—what became known as the refrigerator mother theory of autism—an idea that most American parents and autism specialists had abandoned in the early seventies but that many French specialists had not. (Most have since then.) Lacan's theories, famously difficult to understand, suggested that autism is the psychological result of unconscious parental fantasies that doom their children to be psychic "objects" all their lives, rather than independent "subjects." Touching reinforces this "objectness," so I was reprimanded for tickling the children. There is an adage: "A Frenchman will never let reality get in the way of a good theory." Despite its rich cultural heritage, France has never been known for its open-mindedness; the French will always be the last to accept a new idea, and the last to let it go. Freud said that once he'd won France, he'd have won the world.

Operant conditioning, the procedure we used with Adam, is a concept of the behaviorist school of human psychology, a school of thought that, starting in the late 1950s, began to replace the prevalent psychoanalytic way of thinking about autism.

Behaviorism is based on two important principles, one concerning human psychology and the other concerning scientific process. It argues that (1) all behavior, from the simplest gesture to the most complex lifestyle, exists because it is *conditioned* to exist by the world around us (our parents, rules and regulations, the weather); and (2) any theorizing one engages in should take into account only empirically observable phenomena—things that one can see, smell, touch or hear. (We can't observe joy, for example; we can only observe the laughter that it causes.) Behaviorists, at least the intelligent ones, don't contend that the psyche—the mind as Freud conceived of it—does not exist. They merely contend that since the psyche itself is not observable (it doesn't show up on X rays; it can't be weighed), and since its so-called effects (Freudian slips, dreams) can't be empirically tied to this empirically unobservable source, one abstains from including it in behaviorist theory and practice.

Behaviorism was inspired by Russian biologist Ivan Pavlov's research on animal behavior in the 1890s, but behaviorism as a school of thought in psychology was truly born in 1913, with the publication of John B. Watson's paper "Psychology As the Behaviorist Views It." It made the case for studying how living things (people, for example) behave—why they do what they do—without running the risk of having to speculate on what goes on in their minds, the mind itself being unobservable. Watson, like Pavlov, described behavior in terms of the body's conditioned responses to stimuli. Later B. F. Skinner expanded on these theories by developing operant conditioning, in which a system of rewards and punishments conditions behaviors.

In the 1960s a certain number of psychologists realized that the behaviorist concept of operant conditioning could be applied to the treatment of autistic children, or, more exactly, to their autistic behaviors. Through a rigorous system of reward and punishment, one could teach these seemingly unreachable children not only to sit still, concentrate, speak, refrain from self-injurious behavior and, in general, be more "normal," but to do so voluntarily, without any further reinforcement.

For many years operant conditioning has shown itself to be efficient in modifying the behavior of autistic people. Their "inappropriate" behaviors (rocking, throwing tantrums, not making eye contact, etc.) are targeted to be "extinguished," and specific protocols are set up to accomplish this mission. Every time the person makes eye contact, the behavior is congratulated, positively reinforced, with a cookie, a hug . . . and every time he or she throws a tantrum, the behavior is punished, negatively reinforced: the person is put in a time-out room, scolded, strapped to the chair. . . . It is essential that the specific reinforcements, positive or negative, be tailored to each individual; some autistic people may hate cookies and love being strapped to their chairs. (We all know how reassuring seat belts are.)

(There exist today special helmets conceived for autistic people who bang their heads, bite themselves or tear at their skin. These helmets automatically discharge a small electric shock each time those behaviors occur. Some people find this kind of treatment unacceptable. I myself find it hard to imagine that I actually went so far as to burn Adam S.'s mouth with Tabasco sauce to stop his biting.)

The controversial work of psychologist Ivar Lovaas thirty years ago, early in his behaviorist career, was viewed by some at the time as cruel and extreme (there were rumors that he used strong physical measures as negative reinforcement), but it nonetheless produced undeniably observable and—most important—durable results. His work is represented today by the method called applied behavior analysis, a rigorous forty-hour-per-week, one-on-one operant conditioning program that stresses reward more than punishment.

As systemic and organized as these methods may be, their ultimate efficiency always depends on the quality of the relationship that exists between the person receiving and the person applying the method. Everybody learns better from someone they like a lot; rewards reward and punishments punish in direct proportion to the emotional stakes between the people concerned, autistic or not. Regardless of the results, however, the "normal" behaviors generated by methods like these often remain somewhat robotic in nature: emotionless, machinelike. Recently, more eclectic and interdisciplinary techniques have been put into use in an effort to change this: to permit—or rather to create—emotion and the expression of emotion in the developing autistic child. Stanley Greenspan is one of the principal champions of this movement. He has theorized and described in detail specific ways of playing with autistic children, interacting with them one-on-one ("floor time"—you get down to their level), which he teaches to parents. This technique encourages playfulness, playfulness encourages relationships, and relationships encourage normal behaviors in kids—normal and autistic alike. (Greenspan calls it "emotional learning.") It can be used in concert with various operant conditioning techniques, with other playful techniques that stimulate speech (through picture naming or mime, or through the use of special CD-ROMs that play modified voice sounds which are easier for young brains to process) and with various sensory-integration exercises: massage, skin stimulation (brushing with a stiff brush), various types of visual and oral stimulation and just plain rolling around on the floor tickling each other.

All of the methods mentioned above were conceived with very young autistic children, often starting at one and a half years of age. Their success depends on this early, often massive intervention.

The young Tunisian boy circles around us. He was born in Paris, but he doesn't speak French. He doesn't speak anything. There is no particular expression on his face; his gait alternates between a normal walk and a kind of skipping—he bolts, jolts, jumps forward. It seems that something inside him is exploding, tiny, invisible land mines that go off every ten or twelve steps, each explosion followed by a small moan. He's mined. Someone has booby-trapped this child. Someone or something. Still, for a mine to go off, someone has to step on it, and there's no one around here but us. You can't walk on a land mine that's inside yourself, can you? Or can you? Who's walking on the land mines inside Hakim?

We're standing here talking amongst ourselves: something undoubtedly very important—this year's Beaujolais Nouveau: does it have a raspberry taste like last year, or is that banana? Hakim stares at my forehead. He can't take his eyes off it; his eyes widen. Suddenly like lightning his arm flies forward, his fingers clawed, and as he runs off someone's forehead starts to bleed. The blood trickles down into the person's eyes, blinded now; his eyes are blind now. My eyes.

Hakim does not fit the profile of what we tend to call autism. He is not closed off from the world by an invisible wall; he looks us straight in the eye; he wants to be near us, too near us; his face is expressive; and aside from a few leftover self-stimulating gestures—he stares at the two fingers he holds up to the left of his head, he spins—he does not demonstrate most of the many characteristics of those we tend to call autistic. He seems to understand everything we say as far as simple, common instructions are concerned: go get the plates in the kitchen; put your jacket on; pass the salt—though it's hard to say whether he understands much else: go give Delphine a hug; you should be ashamed of yourself. This is a common problem among nonverbal autistic-type individuals like Hakim for whom IQ tests are not designed.

He bites too. He pounds us on the head; he scratches our eyes; he lacerates our hands (the backs, against the bones where it really hurts); he breaks plates on our heads.

Hakim's clinical history describes a classic autistic child, sequestered within himself, alone in the world, riddled with stereotypical ritualistic behaviors—a child much different from the Hakim that we see today, the Hakim who *won't* be alone, the Hakim who searches us out, finds us, hugs us, hits us. He starts by caressing our foreheads, smiling sincerely, then the smile grows wider as the caress turns into little love taps, the love taps into slaps, the slaps into scratches. He spits in our face and runs away, diabolical laughter ringing in our ears as the blood trickles into our eyes. This Hakim, now twelve years old, seems more psychotic than autistic.

The term "infantile psychosis" is rarely used anymore in the United States. In its place, diagnostic manuals such as the American Psychiatric Association's *Diagnostic and Statistical Manual of Mental Disorders* (known as *DSM-IV-TR*) speak of "Pervasive Developmental Disorders," which include personality disorders, Autistic Spectrum Disorder and, in the case of not-exactly-autism, Pervasive Developmental Disorder Not Otherwise Specified. In France, however, "infantile psychosis" is still employed. The French equivalent of Autistic Spectrum Disorder, this term includes both autism and infantile psychosis—"infantile" meaning beginning in very early childhood, and "psychotic" in this context meaning severely aberrant social behavior, which can include anything from clawing at people's eyes for no apparent reason to reciting Shakespeare to a pair of shoes. The twelve-year-old Hakim described above would probably be diagnosed as having Pervasive Developmental Disorder Not Otherwise Specified, possibly including Personality Disorder.

According to some analytically oriented theorists, the psychotic state is more evolved than the autistic state. The autistic person cannot relate to others; the psychotic person can, but in pathological ways—loving them yet harming them, needing them and destroying what they need in them. These relationships, symbiotic or aggressive, would seem better than no relationships at all; at least you have something to work with. Thus, the autistic child "graduates" into psychosis. If this is true, we ought to be proud that since Hakim's been at our clinic, he has come out of his shell and into our face. Somehow we're not.

I tend to distrust conventional wisdom as a rule, and I distrust conventional wisdom concerning severe psychopathology even more. I do not believe that psychosis is more evolved than autism. I have seen many autistic people become less autistic without becoming psychotic. We lack so much knowledge and reliable data in our business that we can equally argue any position and its opposite. One thing is certain, however: Hakim is dangerous.

I'm sitting on a table in the dining room now. We're in the middle of watching a videotape of a trip we took last year to a horse farm in Brittany, in the west of France. On the television screen we can see Damien, who is attempting to mount a horse for the first time. Everyone claps. I'm clapping, but I'm distracted. Out of the corner of my eye, I see Hakim coming toward me from across the room. I'm not in the mood. He's been hell so far today. The backs of my hands are covered with scratch marks, fresh scabs and open wounds; it hurts to put my hands inside my jacket sleeves. I put my hands inside my jacket sleeves a lot these days. Going out for a cup of coffee down the street, alone.

The dining room rings with applause; Damien just got on the horse again. Big deal. Hakim is halfway to me; he's wearing that smile, the demonic one. I can't do this anymore. I won't look at him. If I don't look at him, maybe he'll go away. An argument broke out in the weekly staff meeting last Monday. Always the same people who whine, *I'm not going to take this! I didn't come here to be bitten and scratched all day long!* I found it incumbent on myself to inform them to the contrary. I presented a dramatic reading from our institution's mission statement, our charter: *"Neither the child's level of violence, nor the scope of his or her inappropriate behaviors, nor the depth of their pathology, may be used as grounds for refusal of admission. . . ."* I explain: Either Hakim is truly diabolical—in which case we must either exorcise or kill him—or he is simply very, very pathological, in which case murder is not a viable therapeutic strategy.

This video horse thing is getting old. I've seen it twice already. (So Damien mounts a horse; I don't see what there is to cheer about.) I'll pretend to be interested anyway, to keep up morale. Now here's Hakim. I won't look at him. I'm not looking. He's climbing up onto the table, sliding up next to me. I work hard at not getting tense—deep breathing, relaxation of the individual musculature through localized meditation, a sixties thing. He's taking my hand, my scab-covered half-bleeding black-and-blue hand. I wait for the nails. I try to remember which of my two hands is more torn up. I won't wince. No wincing. Hakim leaves my hand and takes my arm instead. I knew I shouldn't have worn short sleeves. He's leaning down next to me, on his side. He curls himself up next to me, against me; he takes my arm and puts it around him. Hakim has gone to sleep, his head on my knee. He will sleep there as Damien gets on and gets off the horse, as the video ends and the staff disperses and the other children go home. For some reason my hands don't hurt now. The clinic will close for another day, until tomorrow. And I'm not going anywhere. Until Hakim wakes up, nothing in this world could make me go anywhere else.

In our business we hear lots of stories. The story of the perfectly normal only child who slides into autism after the birth of a little brother or sister. The story of the bright young boy or girl, full of life, who is hospitalized for an ear infection or a tonsillectomy and turns autistic overnight. Hakim's parents say that their son was a perfectly normal baby, and that it was only later, when he was about three years old and found himself replaced at his mother's breast by his newborn baby brother, that Hakim rapidly slid into madness.

If it is difficult to describe what autism "looks like," it seems impossible to know where autism comes from. In the 1950s much of the knowledge about the cause of what was then called infantile autism was based mostly on psychoanalytic—Freudian and post-Freudian—concepts. In general it was assumed (by Bruno Bettelheim, mentioned earlier, for example) that classical autistic behaviors—lack of eye contact, lack of communication, lack of affect (*affect:* expressed emotion)—were in fact psychological defense mechanisms; after some traumatic event or events in very early childhood, however subtle (Mom was having a bad hair day, Baby wasn't quite awake yet), the child "chose" to defend himself or herself against what was experienced as being an intolerable world. This kind of hypothesizing led to a generalized anti-parent attitude on the part of many psychiatric professionals. An awful burden of guilt was laid on the parents of autistic children, and they were often excluded from their child's therapeutic life.

Other psychoanalytic hypotheses were based on the supposition of a "normal autistic phase" of human development, thought to occur in the very first weeks of life, during which the child is shut off from the world by a

27

psychic or psychoneurological "stimulus barrier" that exists to protect the baby from being bombarded by too much sound, sight, smell or touch. A psychological trauma—not necessarily Mom-generated—could cause the child to fixate and stick at this stage, cut off from the world from then on: autistic.

In time better knowledge concerning the psychological profile of the "typical autistic parent" (it turns out there is no such thing) led most people to abandon the "refrigerator mother" theory of autism. Other research concerning the sensory and relational capacities of normal babies has clearly shown there is not, and never was, any such thing as a "stimulus barrier."

For certain psychoanalytic theorists, the breast represents the whole world to the newborn child. Should something go awry during breastfeeding—something real or fantasized (I often wonder: what would a newborn baby's fantasy look like?)—the child may carry the psychological scars with him or her forever.

Melanie Klein, working in the 1930s, thought that the breast, otherwise known as the Object, could be experienced as being Good or Bad according to the relationship that evolves between baby and mother during the first weeks of life. Should this relationship turn out to be complicated or difficult—or should it be experienced as such by one or the other—the baby might feel a certain ambivalence, thus causing him or her to experience the breast as both a Good Object and a Bad Object at the same time, in much the same way that a young child who's hurt himself playing with his favorite windup toy (the spring breaks and hits him in the eye, say) will relate to the toy thereafter with both great affection and great distrust.

Since the mother's breast is so primordially important to the baby, these theorists say, one can easily imagine that this deep-rooted ambivalence could be projected onto other "breasts," other Objects, other people, as the baby grows up.

As a human science professional, I am obliged to maintain a healthy distrust of psychological explanations based on invisible causes and other people's subjective memories. Every day thousands of babies are replaced at their mothers' breasts by younger brothers or sisters without anyone's becoming autistic or psychotic, and though one can always argue that what is traumatic for one may not be traumatic for another, as long as we lack a fact-based description of a coherent selecting mechanism—something that explains *why* what is traumatic for one is not traumatic for the other—simple observation after the fact can carry no real theoretical value.

Hakim is constantly drawn to us, but no sooner does he get close than he is overcome by an uncontrollable urge to attack us and humiliate us, and despite my great skepticism for hypotheses that have no empirical base, it's

29

true: when I look at Hakim pacing back and forth before us, tiny land mines going off inside him, I can't help but see before me a young child of three staring at his mother, stalking her, as she nurses his little brother at the breast that was once his.

Hakim's treatment plan must take into account our weakness as an institution when it comes to dealing with his violence. Some workers can and some workers can't and those who can are few; the notion of teamwork has fallen by the wayside. We feel impotent: our punishments don't punish Hakim. His prescribed medications sometimes work and sometimes don't. We wonder if his parents really administer them at home; they say they do, but their ambivalence about such things has always been clear. (A new generation of extremely efficient psychotropic drugs—therapeutic molecules that calm and stimulate attention at the same time—has changed the face of care for the autistic and psychotic.) But while we have succeeded in finding ways to neutralize Hakim's aggressive drives, our success is always short-lived. Hakim's evolution, or the lack thereof, like that of all our young customers, depends on the quality of our work at the institution as a whole: everything we do or don't or can't; everyone who does or doesn't or won't.

The care plan must be airtight. Hakim is met at the door when he arrives and is accompanied by a member of the staff through every second of every institutional hour (we are an outpatient clinic; we treat twenty customers every day; our clientele arrives at nine A.M. and leaves at four P.M.); he is passed from one caregiver to another like a baton in a relay race. Every activity, every gesture we make, should have an educational or therapeutic reason behind it: to diminish what's gone wrong and enhance what's gone right.

Finding a raison d'être for every minute of every day is exhausting; trying to diminish something we don't understand is killing us all.

Some say that if Hakim doesn't go, the institution will.

Two people on the staff have particularly good relations with Hakim: the cook and the maintenance man. Their natural impassivity has an extraordinarily calming effect on him; they never get scratched, never get bitten. The rest of the staff is full of admiration—or jealous— and so am I. Some have been able to use their example to assume the same demeanor: don't look Hakim in the eye, stay a foot away from him (emotionally as well as geographically), renounce the bleeding-heart sensitivity that people in our business are heir to. The results are obvious. Things go better for them and him.

But for us psychologist types, this raises a question. A certain impassivity on our part helps neutralize Hakim's ambivalence; a reduced demonstration of our emotional investment in him (it's the demonstration that's reduced, not the emotional investment) gives it less to feed on, and allows us to maintain him in a certain state of psychic equilibrium.

But does it *heal*? Does the establishment of a psychological environment where ambivalence cannot flourish cure the patient of his ambivalence? In tri-therapy for AIDS, the virus is rendered impotent by the molecules of the medicines that attach themselves to it. This maintains the patient in good health, but does not eradicate the virus nor cure the patient of AIDS; should the molecules no longer be there, the disease will flourish anew.

The institution suffers from Hakim. His jubilant violence pushes our buttons, our hands covered with scabs that get reopened before they're even closed, our foreheads crosshatched with scratch marks, bruises and teeth marks. We're scared to come to work. Some admit openly that they hate the child and that, ashamed of hating him, have taken to hating themselves. Our center is becoming as pathological as Hakim. We are afraid of where our own inner violence may lead us.

We decide to solicit the aid of a well-known, much-respected psychiatric hospital in Paris that specializes in autism. We ask that Hakim be admitted for a week of evaluation. The idea that our institution is not his last resort is a comfort to us. It relieves the pressure. Without it we won't survive.

We have to wait two months for an appointment. At the appointment, Hakim's urgent hospitalization is scheduled for six months later. Welcome to Paris. When the date finally arrives, we are informed that Hakim will be admitted for day care only and that someone from our clinic must be present half of every day.

In the end the well-known, much-respected psychiatric hospital in Paris that specializes in autism aborts the mission after three days: Hakim is too much for them. The chief of staff allows as how she had underestimated the situation; she promises to reorganize things and readmit Hakim as soon as possible. Two years later we're still waiting. We face the facts: our institution *is* Hakim's last resort.

All mental health workers are not necessarily graced with the specific skills and human qualities required to successfully treat extreme cases such as Adam S. and Hakim. A certain kind of patience is required, a certain form of will and—no, I don't believe it's pretentious to say it—courage. When our institution first opened, I announced to the staff that what we had come together to do there was tantamount to an extended commando mission. They laughed. They're not laughing now.

When one enlists to become a commando, or the member of a SWAT team, one knows what one is getting oneself into. When the chief says, "Men [one supposes such teams are mostly males], we have been assigned a mission that will take us into the depths of the Amazonian rain forest, where we are to rescue eight people who are

33

being held hostage in a tiny cabin surrounded by poisonous snakes and land mines. Statistically it is probable that three of us will die," he doesn't expect the team members to say, "Gee, Chief, I'd love to help you out, but I've got this thing about snakes, see. . . ."

My stance: once one signs on to handle the most severely autistic and psychotic patients—the most dangerous, frustrating, annoying ones—giving up on them is not an option. Giving up one's employment, however, is.

The writing of this book has led me to ask myself many personal questions, the answers to which sometimes surprise me. This one, for example: *No, in the twenty-eight years that I've been working with them, I have never met one single autistic or psychotic person that I didn't like.* (Apologies to Will Rogers.)

Why is this? The writing of this book, I hope, will help me understand.

What are we going to do about Hakim here, in the institution of last resort?

In the 1960s a certain number of new psychotherapeutic techniques were developed in Germany and in the United States. Certain of these techniques were called "regression" or "catharsis" therapy. (Examples are primal scream and rebirthing.) The idea was to enable the patients to relive the painful, deep-seated emotions relating to certain traumatic events in their early childhoods, including birth itself, and in so doing to evacuate them once and for all.

Among these many techniques was a regression therapy called holding, developed primarily by Martha Welch.* In this technique the therapist holds the person in her arms and encourages the person to re-become the baby he or she once was; not simply to remember the traumas of the early months of life but to experience them again, only this time in a situation that is secure and nurturing, as the original situation, apparently, was not. Holding therapy was eventually co-opted and modified for use by psychologists who worked with autistic children. Though it would seem logical that such a method could be applied to help the autistic child overcome the early trauma that supposedly caused him or her to "turn" autistic in the first place—at the hands, perhaps, of a refrigerator mother—such psychodynamic hypotheses about what causes autism had already been left by the wayside in most countries. Holding therapy was put to a different use in the treatment of these children.

One of the more frequent symptoms of infantile autism is the aversion to physical contact. The autistic child cannot or will not tolerate being touched. The version of holding therapy for the autistic concerns training the parents to hold their child in their arms—against his or her will if need be (in principle these are very young

---

* Martha Welch, *Holding Time*, New York: Simon & Schuster, 1989.

autistic children)—regularly, for several minutes at a time. The holding time is then gradually augmented to accustom the child to it. Thus accustomed, the child passes from the acceptance of to the desire for this physical human contact proven (by the early behaviorists, it turns out) to be necessary to good mental health.

Another version of holding therapy with autistics has been developed as a way of extinguishing certain common stereotypical behaviors, such as hand flapping, rocking and head wagging. In this case the parent, trained and supervised by the therapist, physically prevents the child from performing these behaviors: the flapping hands are held still by the parent's hands; the parent prevents rocking by restraining the torso with his or her arms and legs.

Autistic people—Adam S., for example—frequently "explode": they slam themselves against the wall, throw themselves to the floor, they scream, they bite themselves, scratch their own faces, attack anyone in their path. They seem to be quite literally "beside themselves." Sometimes the reasons for these tantrums are obvious. Autistic children are often spoiled: out of indulgent love, or simply to keep the peace, parents tend to refuse them nothing. Then, when it finally comes time to lay down the law, the child's reaction, much like that of a baby (many of these autistic children are mentally retarded) may understandably seem out of proportion. But the cause for such tantruming is often mysterious;

for this reason, many autism specialists have taken a particular interest in the notion of containment. Experience has shown that for autistic people prone to explosion (as opposed to those who are rather apathetic, inert, self-hypnotizing), physical constraining by others—hugging them tightly, for example, using arms as well as legs, "holding" them—can help them learn to "contain themselves."

The most famous example of this is again Temple Grandin. As an explosive autistic child, she could not tolerate being touched. In her memoirs she tells us that she actually longed to be touched—needed to be held—but only in certain exact places and with a certain exact pressure. Though this astonishing woman has overcome her handicap to become a renowned engineer and animal psychologist, she claims that to maintain her psychological equilibrium, she must spend twenty minutes twice a day in her self-designed "hugging machine," a framework box equipped with moving cushions that press on her where and with the pressure she desires.

In France, the John Bost Foundation, a large adult psychiatric facility, has been investigating the notion of containment for many years. When a patient in the male adult autistic unit starts to "explode," six attendants immediately surround him and simply place their hands on him. The calming effect of twelve hands is evident.

In the same vein, the practice of "packing," a technique used in the insane asylums of the early 1900s, has come back into fashion. Violent, volatile patients are asked to lie down on a table, or sometimes in a bathtub, where their individual limbs, their torsos, and eventually their entire bodies are rolled up in cold, damp towels or sheets, preferably in an atmosphere of silence and tranquillity that is often accompanied by nurturing words from the attendant caregivers. With the body thus "contained" by the weight of the wet cloth, its temperature drops, then rises as the body naturally overheats itself, creating a self-generated "heat envelope" that eventually dries the sheets and leaves a sensation of calm and wholeness in the mind and body of the patient. This technique is meant to be applied at regular intervals as a psychotherapeutic protocol. It is not intended for use during the violent episodes.

In our institution we have experimented with several different types of enveloping techniques. A Turkish boy named Osman suffered from a premature adolescence, which started at around age eleven—you could almost see him growing with the naked eye. This drove him to start running into windows, throwing himself against walls, jumping up and down wildly for hours on end and putting on six layers of clothing. Once a week, then, assisted by our nurse, I "mummified" Osman. The sessions began with a systematic body-squeezing massage: starting at the feet, we climbed the legs in eight-inch increments (the width of our two hands), squeezing, then slowly releasing the pressure, inch by inch. We did the same with the arms, then the torso (one of us pushing from behind, the other from in front), and finally the head. These sessions were done in silence; I wanted the effect to be purely sensory, with no intellectual content. Next, we wrapped Osman—feet, legs, arms, torso, hips, head—in long strips of cloth, at first winding them around him loosely, then gradually tightening them as he grew more comfortable with the procedure; and we finished by wrapping wider strips of cloth around his entire body, arms against sides, legs together. We sat with our smiling, serene "mummy" for fifteen minutes, then, very slowly and ceremoniously, we unwrapped him, rolling up the strips of cloth one by one and putting them away as he watched. We took pains to roll them very slowly and very tightly, often using Osman's chest as a table. I came to believe that this last part was perhaps the most important. He was transfixed by it. He seemed to experience the sensation of being mummified all over again, simply by watching, feeling the pressure with his eyes—a visual-tactile sensory double whammy.

In the course of the year, Osman grew steadily less agitated, more "self-contained." He stopped overdressing and acquired a certain stillness, almost poise. These were promising changes, but we will never really know what role our weekly mummifying played in this evolution.

The following year we tried a different technique with an autistic young woman named Liliane. Liliane has no language and is not at all "explosive" (except on rare occasions when, for no apparent reason, she suddenly attacks the person standing next to her, whoever it might be, pulling his or her hair and furiously biting the scalp). Liliane is inhabited by a panoply of hand and arm gestures so pronounced and so constant that it sometimes seems as if her arms are controlling her and not the other way around. These movements are characterized by their omnipresence and by their grace: that of a Tibetan dancer. Frances Tustin, a British psychoanalyst who published in the 1970s and 1980s, divided the autistic into two categories: "confusional" and "encapsulated"—soft and hard.* It's true that some autistic people seem listless, mushy, inert, while others seem rigid, active, electrified. Liliane combines the two—she is fluid and wooden, soft and hard at the same time. What is clear is that these unceasing gestures impede her ability to concentrate and to participate in much of what the world around her has to offer. She is like an orchestra conductor who has conducted so many symphonies for so many years that he is unable to do anything else with his arms.

We tried everything with Liliane—packing, mummifying, holding—but she was too afraid. One look at her face and we would stop. We gradually developed a baroque system involving two big cushions, one placed against

---

* Frances Tustin, *Autistic States in Children*, London: Routledge & Kegan Paul, 1981: ch. 4.

her chest and one against her back, which were squeezed and bound together around her arms and hands by wide strips of cloth: a Liliane sandwich. The effect was immediate. She became still, calm, placid. After a few sessions I took to sitting behind her, gently pulling her to me, encouraging her to lean back at a forty-five-degree angle against my chest. (Up until then Liliane had never been willing to be anything but upright.) This done, I pressed her shoulders together with my elbows while holding her head in my hands. We maintained this position for fifteen minutes, then slowly released everything.

This work did not truly affect Liliane's behavior outside of the sessions. I tried to organize two sessions a day, but the chaotic daily institutional life of mental health commandos made it impossible, a therapeutic luxury we couldn't pragmatically indulge in.

The team of our dance workshop, however, found the time to study Liliane's stereotypical movements; they wanted to learn whether the movements carried content or not. This was done by using dance notation to write movement down on paper, thus allowing a visual "reading" of our Tibetan dancer's exotic *ports de bras*. This reading, when compared with the real-time videotape of what was happening in Liliane's environment, enabled the team to develop a reliable dictionary of her gestures—"Come here," "Go away," "I don't like," "I want to leave," etc.—which would not have been possible otherwise. It dawned on me later that it was just as well that we weren't able to do more containment sessions with Liliane. Their success might have spelled the end to her "speech."

Something has to be done about Hakim. His evil ways have demonized him in the eyes of our staff. Some have gone so far as to postulate that our internal conflicts are a direct by-product of his pathology, that Hakim is in fact plotting to divide and conquer us. The question is hotly debated. Is a mentally handicapped person responsible for the effects of his or her handicap on others? Is Hakim accountable for his violence? We hate cancer, but we don't hate the person who has it. We can say: (1) Hakim *has* a personality disorder that *makes* him behave pathologically, or (2) Hakim *is* a psychopath. The two sentences mean the same thing, but evoke very different responses in us. Arguments over this rage in the institution.

The medieval "possessed by a demon" theory of psychopathology is starting to look pretty good to me about now.

How are we ever going to rid Hakim of his terrible ambivalence—*I crave contact with the people around me, and the moment I get it, I find it intolerable. I love the object and I hate it. I want to be part of it and I want to destroy it, at least humiliate it*—if we can't get around it ourselves?

I devise some tentative hypotheses: (1) Hakim's pathology renders him unpunishable: not only does punishment not punish him, it seems to reinforce the behavior he's being punished for. (2) If this is true, we must admit that operant conditioning does not neutralize Hakim's ambivalence. (3) Which means that we must somehow work "outside" the ambivalent structure. We must create another structure in Hakim, a different, healthy one, in the hope that by its very nature—contentless human affection—it will simply eclipse the ambivalence and take its place.

But how can you create the capacity to love and be loved in the midst of such contradictory emotional drives? We will have to be bigger than they are. And we'll have to start back at the very beginning.

The work will take place in a small room, the same small room every day; the notion of permanence will be essential. The room must be bare, windowless and neutral; in this microcosm nothing must exist except the two of us. Given the precariousness of the mission, I'll need help from the outside—help in keeping myself centered, help in objectively analyzing what happens. One of our psychologists, a psychoanalyst, is free at the hour planned. The work, far from anything Freud ever imagined, will be based on psychoanalytic hypotheses.

Our institution was founded on the principle of interdisciplinarity: all schools of thought—analogous, contradictory, supposedly incompatible—are welcome here. It is entirely possible that Hakim's history as reported by his mother is not faithful to the truth. It is possible that Hakim has never been normal and that the traumatic scene wherein he found himself replaced at his mother's breast by his baby brother never took place, and that his pathology has nothing to do with any of that. But however distrustful I may be of this hypothesis, I say any port in a storm. When we're caught in the tempest that is autism or the kind of "post-autistic psychosis" that Hakim has fallen victim to, any idea, any idea at all, is worth going out of our way for; the stakes are too high. The psychoanalyst will observe us through a video camera installed in the ceiling of the little room. In this room, Hakim's violence, like that of Adam S. twenty-eight years before, not being recognized as such, will not exist. But instead of imitating him as I'd done with Adam S., I have something else planned. In this tiny artificial surrogate world, there will be only unconditional acceptance and tolerance. Perhaps in this way Hakim will be able to psychically restructure himself through the same positive, unconditional physical contact that a baby experiences when held in its mother's arms. A different kind of holding.

I'm already in the room when Hakim comes in, brought here by a caregiver who locks the door from the outside (I have a key, in case). I am sitting in the corner, on the floor. Hakim walks around in circles, exploring. He holds in his hand a large wooden spoon covered with hardened caramel, a vestige from his last activity, our sensory stimulation workshop. I am affectless, neutral, relaxed. I do not look at him. I don't speak. After five or six minutes Hakim starts to get impatient; he wants to leave. He pulls my arm to come open the door. I don't look at him, don't react. He pulls harder, starts whining, gets frustrated. I remain neutral.

Now Hakim explodes—tearing at my hair, scratching at my eyes, biting at my hands, screaming. I block his movements smoothly, mechanically, without looking at him. He backs up, rushes forward, circles around, starts over. At some point, when I sense that he's truly gone out of control, I reach for him and gently pull him down. I wrap his arms around himself, applying the same pressure on his arms that he applies against mine, inch for inch, moment for moment, muscle for muscle. I put my cheek against the back of his head to prevent him from head-butting me. I start to hum an Arabian melody I know, my voice low and open, vibrating against his ear, my breath matching his.

We stay like this, me singing and still, for what seems a very long time. Gradually Hakim starts to relax. I ease my arms. I turn him slightly, let him slip to an angle, and hold him in front of me as a mother would her baby.

Hakim reaches for the wooden spoon he'd left on the floor. He puts it in his mouth and makes a soft, clicking sound, his eyes in middle space. Now he places the spoon in my hand, the bowl against the palm, the handle protruding from between my fingers, then he closes my hand into a fist. Hakim has built a breast. He nurses himself on it. He bites it. He pounds on it with his hand until it falls apart. Then he reconstructs it.

As the session goes on, Hakim leaves the breast intact longer and longer.

I hum an Arabian melody.

I'll spend a year with Hakim in this little room, under the watchful eye of the psychoanalyst. Sometimes Hakim won't want to come. Sometimes, on the contrary, he'll drag me down the stairs. Sometimes he'll be in a hurry to come, then balk before starting. Our sessions take place every Friday, but sometimes on different days of the week he'll come looking for me, pulling at my sleeve to follow him to the little room for a session. He'll run the whole show, putting my arms around him, letting himself go, even falling asleep.

In the room there happens to be a bank of small lockers, some of which contain old files, reams of paper, brochures, plastic balls, rags. Heretofore oblivious to everything but himself and me, Hakim now takes to digging around. On this day he unearths a bunch of old papers (union newsletters). He pulls them out one by one, sniffs them, then crumples them individually, placing the paper balls carefully on the floor. I take his hands in mine, and guide them in picking up the crumpled pieces, in holding them together in his hands, hugging

46

them very tight. I guide him in putting all the crumpled pieces into a little bag that's there. I have him hug the bag. Hakim is hugging the bag, the bag full of crumpled and torn little pieces, holding them together now, reunited. He hugs it in his arm as if it were a baby, his baby, him, in his arms.

Our sessions continue, the school year goes by, Hakim's violence goes significantly by the wayside.

What is inconvenient about psychoanalytic theory is that its hypotheses can be neither supported nor unsupported. This being the case, they may be taken as both ridiculous and miraculous, useful and useless, efficient and nil at the same time. When the young, nonverbal autistic person arrives at the institution angry one morning and his psychoanalyst explains that Antoine is angry because she, the psychoanalyst, was late for his therapy session last week, and when we point out to her that Antoine has arrived angry three days out of five for the last four years, and she answers that the fact that Antoine has been arriving angry three days out of five for the last four years does *not* prove that he did *not* arrive angry today because she was late for his psychotherapy session last week, she is right. As annoying as it may be, her hypothesis, by its very nature, can be neither correct nor incorrect.

In general, it is more interesting to be wrong than to

be right—it makes you search further, learn more. And, strangely enough, bad hypotheses sometimes lead to good ideas.

Hakim takes to scratching himself—under his arms, between his legs. A staff psychologist suggests that, like all newborn children, Hakim is investigating the hinging—the spatial splitting and rejoining—of his body parts: arms that open and close against one's sides, legs that come together and then separate. I don't respond to this. (I think that Hakim has allergies, or maybe crabs.)

Still, it is wise to look longest at what you believe in the least, and as it turns out, I've just gotten an idea. I go to an art supply store and I buy a small wooden mannequin, the kind that has joints—arms, legs, waist, knees, neck—that you can manipulate at will.

Up until now Hakim has treated all objects—blocks, puppets, pencils, dolls—in the same way, as inanimate things: things to put in his mouth, to make piles of, things to bunch together, things to knock apart. Things with no human representation. But the little wooden mannequin will change all that. Immediately, Hakim takes the mannequin in his hands right side up (a rarity), and starts moving him into various human positions. He makes the little man perform a number of feats: taking the chewing gum out of Hakim's mouth and holding it between his little wooden hands, then putting it back where it came from. Hakim lets the mannequin (manipulated by me) tickle and caress him; he even gives the tiny chap a kiss. For the first time in his twelve-year existence, Hakim shows manifest symbolization capacities.

What was wood became alive.

The content of our sessions evolved in step with Hakim's progress. A year later we decided that they were no longer necessary, except on specific, regressive occasions.

The Hakim of today has become punishable, reacting to compliments and reprimands in appropriate fashion. He is calmer and more concentrated, rarely explosive and violent, full of affect and affection. But to this day, when he starts to giggle, we all hold our breath: is this the beginning of a new reign of diabolical laughter and terror? No, it's just the laughter of a boy laughing as all children laugh when they're happy.

Hakim is not cured. The number of severely autistic who are known to have been completely cured can probably be counted on the fingers of two hands. Hakim still becomes aggressive at times—at our center, on the street, at home—but he is no longer a land mine waiting to get walked on. He has good days and bad days, off days and on days. Much depends on who's standing by his side: there are off people and on people; people without and people with patience, courage, will . . . and, say, love.

2

"WHAT BIG EYES YOU HAVE!"
"THE BETTER TO HEAR YOU WITH,
MY DEAR!"

Enghien is a town near Paris known for its gambling casino and its lake, on which, weather permitting, one can canoe. I was there one day, a Saturday, sitting at a sidewalk café with friends and musing about whether people our age could still canoe without looking silly, when suddenly I saw a Beatles song.

I don't think about Beatles songs much anymore. Back when I was thirteen or sixteen, I couldn't get them out of my head. At junior high school I sang in an imitation Beatles group. I still remember the way the girls reacted, screaming as if we were really them, the same girls who'd never given us the time of day before.

Sitting at the sidewalk café in Enghien, I saw a Beatles song in my mind's eye, very clearly. I didn't hear the music; I couldn't think of the words; I had no idea of what its title was.

Here is the Beatles song:

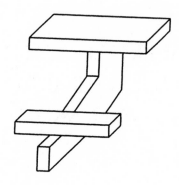

This form, which I had never seen before in my life, came into my head of its own volition. That it was a Beatles song was patently obvious to me. What I did not understand, however, was what there was about it that made it a Beatles song.

(Sometimes when I close my eyes, I see tiny beings. They are animated. Sometimes they are people and sometimes they are stick figures and sometimes they are something in between. They are always in color. They are always very numerous, running around on the floor of a forest. They are different each time; I have never seen them before. Try as I may, I cannot control their movements.)

I drew the form on a paper napkin and showed it to my friends. I said, "This is the portrait of a Beatles song about which I know absolutely nothing."

We canoed.

The next morning, as I was climbing the three steps that led to my girlfriend's door, the lyrics, the music and the title of the song all came to me at once. The song is "Things We Said Today."

"Things We Said Today" is distinguished by its steely strummed acoustic guitar introduction and by the fact that each element of its structure—verse, chorus, bridge— is played in a different style. I learned it forty years ago and can still sing it by heart. The shape that appeared of its own volition in my mind's eye is, beyond a shadow of a doubt, "Things We Said Today."

But why? Why a three-dimensional geometric configuration and not, say, a color? Or an odor? Or a feeling on my skin? What about this form, which can only be perceived visually, makes it the portrait of a song, which can only be perceived auditively? (Leaving aside the question of sheet music.)

One could hypothesize that the two T-shaped parts of the figure which we see facing each other might represent the two *T*s in "Things We Said Today." We could hypothesize that the figure represents two steps, reminiscent of the three steps leading to my girlfriend's door, but though this might explain why the identity of the

53

song was revealed to me on those steps, it in no way explains what about the form makes it "Things We Said Today."

Let's talk about something else.

I know a young man, Alain, who is autistic. His autism falls into the category of "high-functioning." As mentioned before, autism looks different on different people. Many autistic people test out as mentally retarded. One wonders, though, to what extent we can trust IQ and other intelligence tests that were never meant to be administered to such unusual subjects. Putting stock in the results of inquiries and tasks solicited from people who tend to act as if they don't even see you, let alone hear your questions, has always seemed dicey to me. We professionals are constantly being amazed by the seemingly profoundly retarded person who suddenly, quite by accident, starts doing advanced calculus whereas he can't even tie his shoes, or the special-gift genius autistic who can name every subway station in Paris but is incapable of saying his or her own name. In daily institutional life we tend to behave as though every customer (as in "the customer is always right") understands everything we say, but we never count on it.

Alain is thirty years old, comes from a good family, speaks well, has a normal IQ. To the naked eye his stereotypical behaviors seem more eccentric than pathological. When Alain gets bored, which he frequently does, he moves his fingers in a certain way, as if he's doing a cat's cradle with no string. This gesture, he says, makes the time go by. As we've already seen with Temple Grandin, many high-functioning autistic people, as well as those with Asperger's Disorder, a subcategory of high-functioning autism, understand figurative language in a literal way. As far as Alain is concerned, time literally goes by as a result of this finger movement; if he did not move his fingers in this way, he believes, time would actually stand still.

High-functioning autistic people have complex, structured, communicative language (as opposed to those who simply repeat, immediately or afterward, what they hear, a phenomenon called "echolalia"), but it may be otherwise eccentric: in tone, flat on the one hand, weirdly musical on the other, or in syntax, as in "I love popcorn ultimately, very so much!" These people are often capable of becoming autonomous or semiautonomous— taking the subway alone, buying a sandwich, making their bed. Some, not all, of them may also be autistic "savants," possessing special gifts, like the character Raymond in the film *Rain Man* who could calculate enormous numbers instantaneously and memorize complicated statistics at the drop of a hat. Some are able to tell you what day of the week your birthday falls on twelve years from now, or draw in perfect detail the edifice of a Spanish mansion that they saw once, for five minutes, six years ago. (Such gifts, even more amazingly, sometimes appear in low-functioning autistics too.)

People with Asperger's Disorder are almost always autonomous in daily life by the time they are adults. But though they seem normal to the naked eye in every respect, upon further inspection we notice in them a subtle quality, a distance: the "air of aloneness" that Leo Kanner described, the glass wall. This wall may be thicker or thinner from one individual to another, but it is always there. Asperger's Disorder is also characterized by the literal mind-set mentioned above: upon hearing someone described as being "sharp as a tack," the Asperger's person might immediately assume that touching the person in question will result in a puncture wound. But unlike more classically autistic people, those with Asperger's Disorder often learn to control, or at least compensate for, their condition. The fact that many are capable of talking about it also helps.

I know of a case of a severely autistic infant who, thanks to constant treatment by family and professionals for over fifteen years, has grown up to be a normally functioning wife, mother, poet and painter. Though still somewhat eccentric in her manner of speaking and reacting to others, she lives a rich, productive life. Question: Can we say that her autism has been cured? Has her severe childhood autism simply transmuted itself into high-functioning autism? Does she now have Asperger's

Disorder? If so, how did she get it? High-functioning autistic people seem to have normal intelligence levels, though the manifestation of this intelligence, their personal style, may be so eccentric that we don't recognize it as such. Conversely, we may be tempted to attribute superior intelligence to autistic people who don't truly possess it (at least in terms of IQ), so fascinated are we by their originality. Just or unjust, originality is not a criterion for intelligence.

Where do we draw the diagnostic lines? (I would be interested to know where the line is drawn concerning people who experience Beatles songs as three-dimensional geometric shapes and people who don't, for example.) It would be relatively safe to say that high-functioning autistic people still display various symptoms of standard autism, such as insistence on sameness, stereotypical gestures and postures, and occasionally extreme emotional states, whereas the typical Asperger's person tends to present a flat emotional state, almost no stereotypy, and less serious or no obsessive-compulsive behavior.

Alain sees people in a special way. Each human being reminds him of a car—a specific automobile, brand, model and year. Alain also has a personal lexicon. It is made up of invented adjectives that describe the way people are. These words have no semantic roots, no reality-based onomatopoeia (like *choo-choo,* which describes a train), and though Alain can spell his words, it is clear that what's important is not the way the word looks written down. Alain's words are invented strictly for their sound. For example, the word *chatygreaksken* describes "the way the Renault Dauphine was in its time." Alain has informed me that I, too, am *chaty-greaksken*. To Alain my way of being is like a Renault Dauphine.

It seems reasonable that a person's morphology—his or her physical shape—could resemble that of a certain car. How, though, can the vocalized sound of a nonexistent word, with no semantic root or reality-based auditive reference, be used to describe a human being?

No matter; to Alain, the way I *am* is a sound.

To me, the way a certain Beatles song *is,* is a three-dimensional geometric shape.

The golden door that someone like Temple Grandin sees when she hears the words "golden door" is neither a hallucination nor what ordinarily might be called a fantasy. It is a word heard, transformed into an image, *seen.*

Benoit is a nonverbal autistic adolescent with significant intellectual deficiencies. He spends most of his time lying on his stomach, his thumbs in his ears and his fingers in his eyes. When he's not doing this, however, he plays the piano. Benoit employs the two-finger method. His repertoire consists of split two-note intervals played one note at a time. He goes up and down the keyboard, widening and narrowing the interval span at random as he goes.

For the past year, every Friday afternoon a beautiful cello virtuoso has donated her time to accompanying Benoit. She believes that Benoit's playing is not random, that there is reason in the order of his intervals.

All musicians know that the interval called the sixth makes us feel ill at ease, that the seventh makes us feel as if we're on the brink, that the major third resolves the brinky feeling of the seventh and takes us to solid ground, that the major seventh makes us feel romantic. The beautiful cellist is convinced that's where Benoit's pianistics take him and anyone else who cares to listen closely: on a storyless journey through the hilly, heady land of pure emotional sensation.

Benoit also participates in a musical activity led by a jazz saxophone player. (The activity has nothing to do with jazz.) One day last year the saxophone player took to improvising with a long plastic tube that someone had left lying around. He put his mouth on one end, placed the other end over Benoit's ear and started to scat sing, thus introducing jazz into an activity that previously had nothing to do with it. He did this several times. Each time he did, Benoit took his end of the tube and put it against his cheek, then looked into it, wide-eyed.

The saxophone player is convinced that Benoit *sees* sound.

*   *   *

Howard Buten

Several years ago French researchers* conducted an experiment in which autistic children were made to sit in a dark room with earphones on their ears and electrodes on their scalps. Music was played through the earphones; neurosensory activity was monitored through the electrodes. Suddenly a flash of light was produced. The neurosensory monitors indicated that the flash of light temporarily blocked the autistic children's hearing; their audition only gradually returning to normal afterward. The control group of normal children's hearing diminished only slightly after the flash and returned immediately. Soon thereafter a French science magazine's cover read: THE AUTISTIC CAN'T SEE AND HEAR AT THE SAME TIME!

I love science. It's because I do that I tend to believe in scientific data, but not always in the conclusions people draw from them. Decades of daily observations of autistic people do not support the hypothesis that they can't hear and see at the same time. They obviously can. There is, however, another, more general, more intriguing hypothesis to be considered: some autistic people seem to possess a kind of cross-modal sensoriality—their five

* J. Martineau, S. Roux, J. L. Adrien, B. Garreau, C. Barthelemy, G. Lelord, "Electrophysiological Evidence of Different Abilities to Form Cross-Modal Associations in Children with Autistic Behavior," *Electroencephalography and Clinical Neurophysiology,* vol. 82, no. 1 (January 1992), pp. 60–66.

senses intermingling neurologically, superimposing on or replacing one another. This phenomenon is known in some circles as synesthesia.

Damien is a young autistic man who has never spoken a word in his life. He sings all day long, though, his repertoire including themes from popular songs he's heard on the radio or elsewhere, embroidered with his own brand of improvised grunts, roars and trills. (He also does a mean "Ode to Joy" by Beethoven; it came installed on his toy piano.) Like many fastidious autistic people, Damien is extremely preoccupied by the way objects are placed in space—bottles on the shelf, chairs in the hall, pencils on the table, towels on the rack. Objects must be turned in such and such a direction and placed at such and such a distance. Damien cannot stay seated or concentrate on anything unless all the doors within his field of vision are closed. Electrical plugs must be unplugged, and lights turned off during daylight hours. Every time he walks into a room, he rearranges the furniture. He takes anything hanging on the wall off the wall. He scrupulously puts certain items together, pulls others apart. His rigor is impressive, his will absolute.

Years of work—cajoling, insisting, distracting—have attenuated most of Damien's object mania; he can usually get along now leaving things as they are. It's an effort he makes for us. Watching him make this effort is extremely moving.

Becoming a psychologist has not precluded the continued exercise of my two other childhood professions. Thus, I often find myself in theater dressing rooms. Dressing rooms come in all kinds—fancy, plain, tiny, spacious, old-fashioned, modern. With each new theater I discover a dressing room I've never seen before. I begin by walking around in it with my hands at my side, palms out. (I don't close my eyes or chant a mantra; I just walk around.) I feel the space. There are a certain number of things that I have to put in the dressing room: stage makeup (tubs and tubes and sticks of greasepaint, to be placed in their order of application); a small mirror; three violins (full size, small size, miniature); a trumpet; a tuxedo, a shirt, tights, underwear, smock and robe that all hang on hangers; and some hand props. The way to not forget anything is to divide all the items into small groups, each group arranged in exactly the same way every time so as to create a sort of still life, a picture that one gets used to seeing. Anything missing will be sensed— felt, actually, *felt* with my eyes.

As I walk around the empty dressing room I start to decide where things ought to be placed. I move the makeup table, the chairs, the clothes rack, the soap dish, the towels. I open this door and close that one. These choices change radically with each new dressing room I encounter. There are no rules, no empirical reasoning behind my decisions. (Okay, it's true: in winter I tend to put on my makeup near a radiator.) I sometimes come back several times to the same theater. I am sure that I arrange the dressing room differently each time.

What are my decisions based on? What does "feeling with your eyes" really mean?

I know that the objects have been correctly placed in the dressing room by the sensation of well-being that I experience. It is a visceral sensation of muscle relaxation. There is no conscious cognitive element or symbolic explanation involved (I put on the makeup near the radiator because I was weaned too soon from my mother . . .) as far as I can tell. I feel it in my gut.

Does Damien experience the same sensation of well-being when all the doors have been closed, labels aligned and pictures unhung? As long as the doors are open with the labels unaligned and the pictures hung, does he experience a sensation (note that I say *sensation* and not *sense*) of visceral discomfort? Could it be that the same kind of cross-modal sensory superimposition of sight and sound that occurs when a light is flashed also occurs between tactility and sight? Is it conceivable that Damien *feels on his skin* the objects that he *sees with his eyes*?

Sensory perception is not always conscious. We've all had the experience of driving on the expressway and suddenly realizing that, though we've been looking at the road for fifteen seconds, we haven't really been see-ing it. We have been seeing it, of course, but uncon-sciously so. Damien probably doesn't realize why he feels better with the doors closed and the labels aligned. The superimposition of the perceptions involved is likely to be experienced in a subtler, unconscious way, like those of the expressway driver.

Ariel H. is panicking. His morning activity, Circus Skills, is over and the special-ed people want him to go down-stairs—lunch will be ready soon, and they need ten min-utes to put the activity room back in order for the next group. Ariel doesn't want to go downstairs. He won't go. He can't. As if driven by a demon, he takes to mov-ing the gym mats around, stacking them against the south wall—exactly in the middle of the south wall. He puts the rollo-bollos in the closet and closes the door; he lines up the tightwire apparatus parallel to the north wall, exactly parallel, exactly. He is beside himself, sweat dripping off his face, huffing and puffing, gasping for air, wound tight as a rubber band. The staff members are try-ing to explain to him that, this being Wednesday, the gym mats must be carried upstairs to the third floor, where the Relaxation Session will take place at two. As the staff members pull at the mats, Ariel begins to scream at the top of his lungs, pounding them on the back, biting his own hand in frustration, launching his legs against the windowpanes, himself against the wall.

"Listen, Ariel, calm down. It's no big deal. You know that every Wednesday we loan the gym mats to Helène and Christianne for their Relax—"

But it *is* a big deal, a very big deal indeed, to Ariel H. You would say that his life depended on it. It takes three staff members to pull him out of the room, lock the door and hold him down on the hallway floor.

I show up (I'm definitely never going to get the County Mental Health report out by noon). I hold my hand up, elbow bent, the Native American sign for *ugh*. "Unhand that man!" I want to say. "What's this all about?" comes out instead. I take a step forward, do the breaststroke with my arms (the Native American sign for "Unhand that man"). They unhand Ariel H. I unlock the door to the circus room. He runs in and immediately sets about rearranging the mats and the tightwire, the inner tubes and the trampoline, the rollo-bollos and the stilts. He calms down, left to his own devices. He inspects his work, checks it twice and walks out the door and down the stairs to the dining room.

Lunch went fine. Veal chops.

Franck L. belongs to the elite club of non-high-functioning autistic savants mentioned earlier. Although he speaks with great difficulty, if you give him the date of your birthday and any year, past or present, he will immediately tell you what day of the week it fell or will fall on. He loves to do it.

(Oliver Sacks, the famed neurologist, having studied a small group of autistic savants, came to the conclusion that they "see" the dates in their head, scattered in a sort of mental landscape, and need only to look around a little to see the day of the date. This hypothesis, which is far from being corroborated, will be of interest to us in the coming discussion.)

Franck is a tall, stocky, teenage butterball with an awkward air and a labored step. He speaks slowly and must repeat every phrase several times if uninitiated listeners are to understand him. One day as we were walking down the street together, Franck suddenly stopped on the sidewalk. Staring into middle space, he began pronouncing what appeared to be isolated single words. I was able to understand many of them, but could make no sense of the whole. It was only when I turned around to continue our walk, and noticed the poster taped to a lamppost behind me, that it dawned on me that Franck had been reading it aloud. I took to pointing to the words and asking Franck to read them individually, out loud. He did this easily for most of the words, but drew a blank on others. I realized then that he couldn't exactly read, that he'd never learned to "sound out" words, but that he'd simply memorized a number of words—an incredible number, it turns out—as "drawings-with-a-name," neither distinguishing the sounds of their individual letters (he can, however, spell them out loud) nor necessarily understanding their meanings (though usually he does).

A couple of years ago Franck started manifesting strange behaviors. He would put his ear against the wall (or against a radiator or a windowpane), wait for what would seem to be a calculated number of seconds, then pound the surface beside his ear with the heel of his hand, two quick hits, like a doctor thumping a patient's chest and back, sound-checking for congestion. He goes into any and all rooms—he comes and asks us to unlock them if they are locked—puts his ear to their wall and knocks twice. This sort of manic strangeness—these autisms—are thought by some to be behaviors that need extinguishing. I, however, put myself in his position and immediately realize the comfort that this brings to Franck. Until I fully understand what he is comforting himself *against,* I will continue to open all the doors of all the rooms whose walls are worth thumping.

I know the feeling. . . .

Like everybody else, I believed when I was young that there were monsters in my bedroom closet. Like everybody else, I knew that they moved elsewhere during the day, and came back, monstrously, after nightfall. (This was in accordance with the Closet Monster Mobility Act of 1953.)

To ensure proper closure of one's closet, it is necessary to push on the doorknob. Logic dictates that if pushing on the doorknob ensures proper closure of the closet door, pushing *twice* on the doorknob should ensure its proper closure twice over; three times, thrice over, etc. By the time I was five (the most reasonable of all ages), I found myself standing nightly at the closet door, pushing on the knob fifty times before I could, in all good conscience, even consider going to bed.

Anyone who was ever five knows how time-consuming pushing on doorknobs fifty times can be; one is far too busy to indulge in such security-driven strategies, however necessary they are. Preoccupied by the idea of efficacy (and the need for some shut-eye), I decided one day that simply touching the doorknob was tantamount to pushing. So each night before I turned the bedroom lights out then, I would stand there and touch the doorknob fifty times, rapidly, counting out loud through breathy inhalings and exhalings, before jumping into the sack.

As was Einstein's General Theory of Relativity in 1915, the proof of this method's efficacy was confirmed a year or two later when I was able to declare that in all my years of doorknob touching, I had never, not even once, been killed and eaten by a monster.

What is pertinent about the closet story is not that I had convinced myself that there were monsters inside. What is pertinent is that I convinced myself that touching the doorknob lightly and repetitively with my finger was the equivalent of pushing on it hard with my hand, in spite of the fact that such a deduction was in no way coherent with my everyday experience nor with my theretofore acquired knowledge. And yet I truly believed that should my hypothesis be wrong, it would cost me my life.

What is also pertinent here is that I never bothered to question this hypothesis, though at the time I questioned *everything,* as did Einstein, my hero even then.

Whenever I lie down on a mattress for the first time, it takes me a moment to feel at ease. To feel at ease, it is often necessary that I shove the pillow a little this way, plump it up a little that way, try this side of the bed and then the other, spread myself out at various angles within the rectangle of the frame, in much the same way as I am driven to arrange and rearrange the various objects in unfamiliar theater dressing rooms.

Bedding is complicated. The innate particularities of a mattress—too soft, too hard, listing to the right, sagging to the left—are already difficult enough to control; the peculiar geological inequities of the feather, cotton or foam stuffing are enough to drive the sensitive sleeper mad. Mattresses necessarily have highs and lows, nooks and crannies, hills and dales. These topographical details may be invisible to the naked eye, or not immediately perceptible to our innate tactile sensory equipment; most sleepers don't even notice or, if they do, don't care. Others do.

Though the two states of mind and body always function in concert, it is important to distinguish between *hypersensitivity* and *sensory preoccupation*. Hypersensitivity is reactive: in a world with zero sensory stimulation, hypersensitivity does not exist. Sensory preoccupation, however, is active, like radar. It is there, ready, waiting for the next odor, temperature change, itch, sound, visual effect . . . or mattress lump.

I believe that there exists in certain people a special psychological state, situated somewhere between the intellectual knowledge of the physical composition of things—real or imaginary—and how they act and react, and the physical sensations—necessarily real—that the composition, action and interaction of these things provoke in us. (All physical sensation is necessarily real and current, even if its source is not. Everyone knows that the simple imagining of chewing on ice cubes gives us physiologically real shivers.) This psychological state is what I call sensory preoccupation. The difference between being "sensorially preoccupied" and simply "sensing" is that the former term includes the notion of attention—of *willfully* being open to, though not necessarily searching for, sensory experience.

I'm lying in bed in my hotel room and I'm slightly uncomfortable, due to the hills and valleys in the mattress. I decide to equalize the surface of the mattress by pulling up on the valleys and pushing down on the hills. This takes a certain amount of time, but in the end I get the job done. Comfortable at last, I turn the lights off and lie down. But now, in the dark, I realize that I am not at ease in the bed; I feel that something is skewed— unequal, akimbo. I reach my arms out horizontally to touch the edges of the mattress and I ascertain that I am closer to one side of the bed frame than to the other. I slide myself toward what I perceive to be the middle of the mattress according to my outspread arms, the hands on the end of which are still touching the frame. Yet something is still wrong. I reach up and turn on the light, look down at myself and observe that although my larynx— the point equidistant between the ends of my two horizontally outstretched arms (assuming that my arms are of equal length)—is exactly equidistant from the two borders of the bed frame, the majority of my body— everything below the collarbone—though perfectly in line with itself, is lying at a slight angle relative to the rectangular edges of the bed.

When I am on tour, every new night brings a new bed with new hills and new valleys, and other lumps and various crests, night after night, bed after bed. My tech crew never complains about their mattresses. They never seem to notice any nooks or crannies. They start talking behind my back. I hear shrouded references to the Princess and the Pea.

The process of Serta-perfect lump control becomes a ritual, a preventive measure to be executed before bodily entering the rectangular bed-space, as does the regulatory process of verifying the geometric centering of one's *self* within the bed-space relative to its parameters.

In time I find myself going through the motions every night, from the moment I enter the room, even if the mattress turns out to be lump-free, and my body dead parallel center. Going through the motions takes only a minute; it can't hurt.

The above anecdote is for the most part fiction—I do not spend my time pinching and punching bedroom equipment. Though I am sensitive to unevenness in mattress surfaces and proximity to borders, I do not allow myself to be obsessed by such things. The reason is simple: I have other, more important things on my mind. (Sleeping, for example.) The autistic do not. They do not have the same preoccupation with getting enough sleep that you and I have. They do not lead the same lives that we lead. Autistic people have not been socially conditioned to believe that such things as mattress punching are simply *not done,* largely because, given their innate, undoubtedly hardwired preoccupations, there is no reason, logical or visceral, that they should be so concerned.

Having no greater preoccupations, Franck senses the air that fills a room as being riddled with hills and hollows (as it probably is), in the midst of which he feels uncomfortable. His strange arm gestures give him the feeling that he has rearranged the air, or at least had some effect on it (which he undoubtedly has), thus allowing him to feel more comfortable in it, which he does. That he does proves that his method is efficient, in the same way that my method of ensuring the closure of my closet door—tapping on the doorknob fifty times with my finger—was proved efficient.

These acts serve to make us feel that we are in control of a situation more than they serve to solve an actual, material problem. That the closet door in the end is more closed than before or not, or that the air molecules in a room are more tolerably dispersed or not, matters little. As is usually the case in daily life, it's how we make ourselves feel that counts. Though these feelings are by definition subjective, they are soundly based on observable phenomena. All observation is sensory—a hallucination is perfectly observable to the person who

hallucinates—and each individual has his or her particular set of sensory aptitudes and preoccupations.

Unlike me with my closet-closing technique, however,
the autistic do not, I believe, feel the need to justify their
ritualized actions—either to others or to themselves. I
do not believe that Franck tells himself, "I sense that the
air over here is too thick, and that the air over there is
too thin, and since this is putting a crimp in my evening,
I'm just going to push these molecules over here farther
over there [gesture]. Fine. Now I can go in and stare at
this pile of magazines that I carry around all day for a
reason that no one in this institution can understand."

When our nose itches, we just scratch it; we don't explain it to ourselves.

Autistic gestures are fascinating. They are totally original and perfectly mysterious. Why this exact movement
and not another? It is often said of these movements that
they remind us of the religious in prayer—the torso rocking back and forth, the head bobbing—or of whirling
dervishes who spin in circles, thus achieving a state of
divine dizziness. What, we might wonder, makes this
dizziness divine instead of, say, nauseating? Studies done
on joggers suggest that repetitive strenuous movement
tends to raise the levels of beta-endorphin in the brain,
inferring that the autistics' rhythmic, strenuous movements serve the same purpose. (Try rocking back and

forth from the waist for ten minutes in a sitting position; you'll understand. . . .) Beta-endorphin, as mentioned before, is an endogenous opiate—"opiate" as in *opium*— and as it happens, it is found not only in the brain but elsewhere in the human body (for example, in the gut). Since it acts as a natural analgesic, or painkiller, one could imagine that the autistic person came upon these rocking or spinning movements accidentally one day and, given their particularly pleasant effect, took to repeating them often. (They are cheaper than whiskey and more legal than pot.) Since, as noted, research shows that many autistic people already have elevated levels of beta-endorphin, this would explain their resistance not only to pain but to extreme temperatures. (Rare is the autistic child who bothers to put on a coat before running out into subzero weather and staying there.) This finding is not in contradiction with their instinctive efforts to obtain more, as any self-respecting alcoholic or avowed pothead knows.

(As I write this, certain autism researchers are starting work with pharmaceutical laboratories in an effort to develop diagnostic markers for autism based on analyses of blood and spinal fluid; elevated levels of pentapeptides, such as beta-endorphin, are among the primary marker candidates.)

It is often said that the autistic use their stereotypical gestures to cut themselves off from the world around them. I don't necessarily attribute such causal reasons to these gestures. It is true that while a person is busy staring at something, or rigorously rocking back and forth, he or she is less attentive to other things. But I do not believe that the autistic shut out the world on purpose, any more than the multinational CEO does as he talks incessantly into his cell phone to the exclusion of everyone and everything around him.

Other stereotypical gestures are more difficult to understand; certain hand movements, for example: flapping one or both hands in front of one's eyes or to the side of the head, and staring at them for long periods of time. These behaviors would seem to fit into the "hypnotic" category. The true neurological action of hypnosis is not known (especially when it comes to the matter of posthypnotic suggestion), but one may assume that processes similar to those of rocking may be at the bottom of these activities. If we believe in the hypothesis of sensory cross-modality, we might imagine that staring at one's flapping hands (hands "rocking back and forth" rapidly) might produce the same neurological effect that bodily rocking back and forth does, the proprioceptive neurological pathways superimposing on, or crossing with, the visual pathways. (Proprioception is the sensory feeling of the position of one's own body from the inside.) Other autistic hand movements remain mysterious: the ritualistic tensing of certain fingers, the peculiar curving inward or outward of the palms, the staring at them. I often wonder if the hand configurations in question don't serve as small sculptures, held up for study in the same way that a painter continually steps back to examine his or her last brush stroke, considering the light and how the canvas itself looks set off against the background of whatever objects or windows happen to be in the studio at the time.

Staring at your fingers held to the side of your head produces the pleasantly painful sensation that comes from pushing the eye muscles to their limit. (It's like a cat's stretching, only it's your eyes.) At the same time you can savor the sensation of focusing alternately on the foreground and the background. In the backseat of the car, you can make the little smudge on the window hop over the treetops or houses passing by on the highway, instead of just sitting there being bored.

It would be fascinating to film the gestural history of an autistic person as one films the life's work of a choreographer or painter.

What does it mean to say that someone "performs a certain gesture one day by accident"? What does it mean to say that when your nose itches you simply scratch it without explaining it to yourself? Actions like these do not qualify as reflexes. A reflex is involuntary. Scratching one's nose, like flapping one's hands and staring at them, is not a reflex. Yet we assume from personal experience that autistic persons do not say to themselves: I think I'll just flap my hands in front of my eyes and stare at them for a while, because when I do this I always get a nice buzz. . . . Ah, there, that's better! What *do* autistic people say to themselves about their gestural behavior? If they don't say anything to themselves about it—that is, if they don't "think" about what they're doing and if what they're doing does not qualify as reflex—then what *is* it that they're doing? How exactly do they come to do what they're doing? By what process? Cognitive psychologists speak in terms of "action plans" and the notion of "intentionality." Two people playing catch go through a seemingly infinite number of eye-hand coordinating steps and muscular adjustments to get the mitt where it has to be to stop the ball in mid-flight. Yet these steps are not thought through in the sense that one thinks through a decision before making it. One doesn't "cogitate" on how to get the glove to where the ball will be.

What *is* intentionality?

I'm sitting in a friend's house, watching television, getting bored. Without thinking, I start to beat out a funky rhythm on my knees (remember, I used to be a drummer). The rhythm is complex, syncopated and dynamically varied. I wail. It takes me a few minutes to realize (very consciously) that I never *decided* to beat out this particular rhythm; I didn't have it ready in my head, nor had I been grunting it internally at any time during the day. I did not go "and-a-one-and-a-two . . ." leading up to the first hand slap on my knee. I have no idea why I am beating my knees to this beat and not to one of the other three-hundred-odd beats that I could be beating my knees to.

What mental process is at work here?

Cognitive science today is faced with the challenge of explaining and articulating complex, subtle and *hypothetical* neurophysiological processes without having anywhere near the empirical cellular, biochemical and anatomical data necessary to do the job. Lacking these facts, these scientists invent constructs that serve as conceptual substitutes: Reciprocal Facilitation, Chaining, Corollary Discharge and Ecologically Dynamic Sub-Persons. This field of research speculates on the possible relationships amongst perception, sensation and motor command. Given what we know about the curiously elaborate and special relationships many autistic people seem to have with these three areas of psychological functioning, it behooves us to follow this research very closely.

Many autistics demonstrate a peculiar sensorimotor need to control their environments. According to my own hypotheses, neither is this a matter of hallucination nor is it one of imagination (as was my need to control the monster-in-the-closet situation in my bedroom). The intolerable—or at least very annoying—environmental elements that engender the extravagant air sculpting, furniture moving and self-winding and -unwinding in the autistic are experienced by them sensorially as real. For that very reason they are, as the following findings show.

R. I. Birdwhistell,* a nonverbal-communication specialist, demonstrated that a person's skin vibrates subtly to the sound of the voice of someone speaking to him. Recent experiments indicate that the viscera—the internal gut organs—may actually operate as a second central nervous system. Certain hypotheses concerning the existence of "cellular memory"—local skin cells that "remember" and react to an old wound without participation from the brain—are being considered anew. Studies by Margaret Bauman, a Boston neurologist, suggest that there exists an "associative" area in the brain, particularly developed in the autistic, in which separate pathways from separate senses may interact, superimposing on one another, mixing with one another, canceling one another out.

Research, if it's done right, should raise more questions than it answers.

What would Temple Grandin see in her head if Alain asked her to imagine someone who was *chatygreaksken*?

What would Alain answer if he were asked to describe the way a Jackson Pollock painting is?

What would Damien do if he found himself in an

* R. I. Birdwhistell, *Kinesics and Context: Essays on Body Motion Communications*, Philadelphia, Pa.: University of Pennsylvania Press, 1970.

empty room with holograms of open doors projected on all the walls?

And you? If someone were to ask, "What does the song 'Things We Said Today' look like?" how many of you would reply,

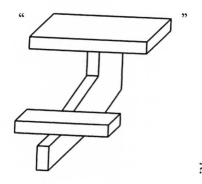

?

3

APPLES AND ORANGES

In 1985, my internship completed, I left the institution in the southern suburbs of Paris where I had been sanctioned for imitating and tickling the patients. This remains the worst professional experience of my life. It took a Herculean effort to finish out the year there, licking my wounds and gritting my teeth (two things very hard to do at the same time). It was only several years later that I realized that I had gotten what was coming to me. Every institution has the right to decide which theoretical bases and practical guidelines it wishes its workers to follow. Though I had more years of experience than the director herself, I was still only an intern, and as such had no business swimming upstream in a workplace to whose theories I could not adhere.

I had been told that in imitating the autistic I was

showing them, and I quote, the "Face of Death," though proof to the contrary had already been well documented.*

In 1989, wounds licked, together with an actor/ musician colleague who ran a brilliant theater activity in the institution mentioned above, I created a one-day-a-week, wild and woolly, y'all-come, one-hundred-percent-volunteer recreation center for the autistic of all ages. It was named Koschise; my French colleague was not gifted in spelling the names of Apache Indian chiefs. Every Thursday from two to four P.M., we received fifteen or so autistic people of all ages in a condemned house behind a post office, and painted, sang, danced, massaged, rapped, hopped, skipped and jumped with them. (Recently the colleague, who has since become a university professor in communications, reminded me of how three or four of us would occasionally take a severely autistic teenager or two and set them free in a shopping mall to observe them; we'd peer around corners and hide behind columns, studying their free-roaming public behavior, as well as the reactions of the normopaths and salespeople who encountered them.)

At that time I also went to work every Thursday at a different kind of outpatient clinic called an *hôpital de*

* The book *Sonrise*, by Barry and Fran Kaufman, published in the late 1970s, tells the story of how countless hours of imitation led their son, Raun, to a full recovery from autism.

jour, a day hospital, which had an adolescent and young-adult autistic clientele. Learning of my travails at the previous institution, and being themselves at the forefront of the long overdue backlash against the French psychobabble establishment, my new psychiatrist colleagues invited me to pursue my research on imitation and empathy, using youngsters from Koschise as well as from the *hôpital de jour* to participate with me in twenty-minute videotaped imitation sessions. These were to go on for many months. Our intent, far from being rigorously methodological, was simply to see how the various participants took to being locked in a room with a foreign weirdo who did everything just like them. The sessions with a certain Ramdan, a sixteen-year-old nonverbal autistic Moroccan, were particularly spectacular. Ramdan loved to be imitated: every gesture, every sound drove him into ecstasy. Our sessions evolved into incredible gibberish rap competitions, ever wilder, louder, more extravagant with each turn. The same went for our nonverbal exchanges. Ramdan puts a cushion on his head, Howard puts a cushion on *his* head; Ramdan puts a book on the cushion on his head, Howard puts a book on the cushion on *his* head; Ramdan puts a stuffed bear on the book on the cushion on his head, Howard puts a stuffed monkey (we were out of bears) on the book on the cushion on *his* head. Ramdan puts a bowling ball . . .

In the course of the project, I started straying from the

protocol. It had been understood that I was to "mirror" my partners, do exactly what they did as they did it, but after a while I instinctively wanted to become like them in general—act just as they acted, assimilate and reenact their exact repertoire of behaviors, but not necessarily at the same time or in the same order.

Though no statistical analysis was employed, it was clear that becoming autistic in the fashion of the person with whom I shared space rendered me more interesting to them than would otherwise have been the case. As with Adam S. sixteen years before, the special relationships initiated in the imitation room between me and my extravagant partners in mime spilled out into real life, insofar as the goings-on at an *hôpital de jour* can be deemed real life.

The project at the *hôpital de jour* had come on the heels of another, similar study that I'd done in 1986 at a very different kind of institution.

Given my tarnished French reputation in the south Parisian suburbs, I was flattered when the chief of staff at a large psychiatric facility only a mile away invited me to speak to the clinical personnel on the topic *empathie: une passerelle vers des relations d'objets affectives chez l'enfant autiste nonverbal.* ("Empathy as a Bridge to Affective Object Relations in Nonverbal Autistic Children: A Psychodynamic Theory" was the title of my doctoral dissertation.)* The word of my imitating, for better and for worse, had gotten around fast. At the end of my lecture the chief of staff approached me. "Have you ever thought of trying out your ideas on an older population?" he asked.

In those days everyone was still associating the word *autistic* with children—autistic children—myself included.

"I'd love to," I said. "How much older are we talking about?"

He stared at me.

"Much," he said.

Le Centre Hôpitalier Spécialisé de Perry Vaucluse is a sprawling psychiatric facility (1,406 beds) on the outskirts of Paris. My research is to take place in a certain pavilion that had been built between the two world wars as a temporary one-story structure. You can tell it hasn't changed a bit; it looks like a prefab school left over from the fifties. Immediately there's The Smell, the one I will never again wholly get out of my nostrils, the unique aroma that permeates such places, that has been permeating them since the Middle Ages. Asylum Number Five. I enter from the front, pass by a small guardian's cubicle and continue through the TV room. Suddenly I find myself standing before a mammoth green wall. Its door has

---

* The Fielding Institute, Santa Barbara, California, 1985.

the biggest lock I've ever seen. Stretched across the wall, full width and six feet off the ground, is a narrow row of windows. I try to look in but I'm not tall enough (I'm five foot eleven and a half), so I stand on my tiptoes. Through the window I see a huge, bare room with wooden benches running lengthwise down each side and nothing else. Nothing, that is, besides fifteen naked or nearly naked men—eighty years old, fifty years old, thirty-five years old; toothless, ageless, nameless; rolling on the floor, staring at their fingers, talking to themselves in a corner, crouched motionless with their hands around their heads. In the very back (my legs are beginning to cramp from standing on my tiptoes, but I can't take my eyes off what I've been smelling), I see white-tiled stalls in which nurses are hosing down the naked men one at a time.

The pavilion is named Ventose (*vent* means wind, as in "ventilator")—the old French name for the windy sixth month of the republican year (*année républicaine*, the calendar created after the French revolution; part February, part March). Divided in two sections, Ventose serves as lodging for some forty men, half of them mentally retarded, half autistic. Their mean age is sixty. The patients in the retarded section (one doesn't say "intellectually challenged" in France; never did, never will), most of whom have Down syndrome, sleep in bedrooms, alone or two together. They all wear sweat suits, and they spend their days in the TV room, in the yard or in the hallways between their rooms. The autistic patients sleep together in a large hospital ward. They spend their days in the huge locked dayroom or occasionally, for a few hours, in the yard. Naked or in open-backed hospital gowns until lunch, they are clothed for the rest of the day in sweatpants, hospital gowns and house shoes—the same faded plaid felt house shoes that you will find in all, absolutely all, psychiatric hospitals in France, and that you will never, ever, *ever* be able to see again—in job-lot stores or Salvation Army shops around the world—without your nostrils filling mysteriously once again with The Smell.

I have never felt more at home.

Few people from the outside ever set foot inside the autistic section of the pavilion. The interns I meet from other pavilions tell me that no one has ever even mentioned the place to them in the months since they arrived to begin their year, though they are aware of it. They say the nursing staff of Ventose is infamous, widely renowned even in the farthest corners of the hospital for its meanness: they will chew you up and spit you out. Thus warned, I walk trembling into the long clapboard building, hat in hand, to unveil my project to the evil staff.

It takes me all of five minutes to realize that I have indeed happened onto a highly unusual team of nurses. They are extraordinary. Tough on the outside to all those who do not dare venture into the netherworld of the Windy Pavilion—those who don't even have the professional curiosity to come and see—they are prepared to move heaven and earth for the care and well-being of their men.

I have found clinical heaven.

Our project will consist of individual sessions, twenty minutes long, three times a week, with three of the autistic men. During these sessions, I will imitate them— "become" each of them in much the same way that I would become Ramdan and two other young autistics at the *hôpital de jour* three years later. The sessions will be taped by the nurses. These tapes will be analyzed by those interns to whom no one had ever mentioned the existence of this pavilion (I don't believe a word of it), using grids I've prepared which indicate the frequency of reciprocally imitated behaviors—them imitating me imitating them—and that designate signs of affective relations: smiling, coming close to me, touching or making significant eye contact with me and the like.

The room to be used is, in fact, a space in the back hallway of the building, curtained off with hospital bedsheets pilfered from a locked closet. I am surreptitiously sneaked one of each article of clothing worn by the patients (one hospital gown, a single pair of jogging pants, a sweatshirt and a pair of house shoes). The protocol specifies that I already be in the room when each subject arrives, behaving like him, dressed exactly as he's dressed.

To ensure that the study is done under the most rigorous conditions (studies of this kind never really are), I will have to select three subjects, all of whom not only are autistic but also demonstrate the same kinds of autistic behavior: a homogeneous test sample.

Since each of the subjects is to perceive me as being autistic and similar to himself, it will be necessary that they not see me anywhere other than in the experimental setting. To this end the very first thing I do, to the general hilarity of the staff, is put on the hospital gown and jogging pants and those felt slippers and slide unnoticed into the dayroom, where I perform a wide gamut of autistic behaviors—a composite of four or five former patients I'd particularly admired, classic cases, a sort of autistic "best of."

As it turns out, I am so involved in my role of Autistic Person Cut Off from the World that I'm incapable of noticing what my co-autistic neighbors are doing. Thus, I am obliged to rely on the nurses to choose my three subjects—to arrive at a consensus concerning which three are the most alike. To make things easier, I offer to make a checklist of behavioral criteria. To guarantee the rigor of the profile I am looking for, and in the interest of scientific process, I produce a list even more detailed and explicit than the one found in the standard psychiatric resource of the time—the third edition of the *Diagnostic and Statistical Manual of Mental Disorders*, otherwise known as *DSM-III*.

Here is my list:

Howard Buten

DIAGNOSTIC CRITERIA
FOR INFANTILE AUTISM*

- air of aloneness
- does not react when called
- avoids eye contact
- resists changes in the environment
- seems uninterested in what's happening around him/her
- uses people as objects (example: uses someone else's hand instead of his or her own)
- absence of, or strange quirks of, language (pronomial reversal, blabbering, echolalia)
- demonstrates stereotypical gestures: hand flapping, rocking, staring, nodding, finger twiddling, etc.
- walks on tiptoes
- is self-injurious: head-bangs, self-bites, self-scratches, etc.
- has normal physiognomy
- may demonstrate exceptional intellectual/fine-motor skills: memorization, calculation, drawing, date naming, etc.
- demonstrates attention deficits
- flat affect (talks or moves like a robot)

---

* The current *DSM-IV-TR* uses "autistic spectrum disorders," a broader term that encompasses a wider range of presenting symptoms, and thus more people who fit it. Back in 1985, "Infantile Autism," the term coined forty years earlier by Leo Kanner, was still the term of choice.

(*Note:* Given the age range of our subject pool and the impossibility of verification—most of their original files having been lost, or being so old and decrepit as to be unreadable—I omit the standard criterion: "Onset of symptoms before three years of age.")

Most of the men in the autistic wing of the Ventose pavilion seem clearly to be autistic. If they weren't when they first came there, they have certainly grown into it since; the vast majority of them have already been here for at least forty years, and the phenomenon of "acquired stereotypical behaviors" in mental hospitals is well-known.

It will take three meetings and dozens of hours for us—the nurses, the nursing supervisor and me—to finally come to an agreement about which three men are the most similarly autistic. ("He does not avoid eye contact!" "Yes, he does!" "Does not!" "Does so!") It comes down to a certain Baba (thirty-seven years old), a certain Lekbir (forty-two years old), and a certain Little Joe (fifty-five years old)—not to be confused with Big Joe, another patient, who is younger than Little Joe but much larger. Thus assured of the homogeneity of my sample—a homogeneity determined by my own, very detailed, written criteria and the consensus of opinion concerning its interpretation by the hospital staff of seven professionals (I will come back to this)—we begin the first day of sessions in the following order: Baba, Little Joe, Lekbir.

Baba is tall and very thin, with dark hair. He is dressed in a hospital gown, open in the back, and sweatpants. He rocks back and forth on his feet, his arms always out in front of him, elbows bent and at different angles, fingers stretched and twisted into strange forms, like knotted, tortuous vines. He says only "Ba . . ." or "Baba . . . ," his cheeks puffing and releasing; he pauses regularly to hold a twisted hand up to his eyes and stare at it, sometimes for up to a minute, then returns to his rocking. Sometimes he shakes his hand as if it were a tiny whip, or as if he were attempting to shake off a ladybug that's perched there and won't leave. He won't look at me . . . suddenly he stares at me . . . then he won't look at me. From time to time he takes one of his hands in the other, squeezes it, the thumb of one hand pressing down in the palm of the other, and stares.

It is very comfortable to imitate Baba (I am told that his real name is Maurice, though no one has called him that in twenty years). He has great blue eyes, and when he sets them on me and stares, it becomes obvious how taken he is by the fact that someone else is rocking like him and talking like him. I take pains to keep my *Ba*'s in the same key as his, and I use the same tone, that of a clucking chicken. Thus I am able to inspire him to imitate me in return—imitate me imitating him: I squeeze my palm and he immediately follows suit; he is silent until I start *Ba-ba*-ing, then he joins in the refrain.

Little Joe is dressed in the same way as Baba. This man of fifty-five years, hospitalized here all his life, will do nothing—literally nothing—but swivel back and forth on his legs, as if his whole rigid body were a half orange on an old-fashioned juicer, stuck in endless instant replay, pushing himself down and swiveling long after all the juice is gone. His head, also stuck, is turned to look over his left shoulder, but his eyes are closed. Occasionally he will open them into slits—one second, two—then close them again. The only other gesture he ever makes is to flick his lips with his thumb, then hold the thumb aside, then flick again . . . and again . . . and again.

Lekbir is supple, almost graceful. He is dressed in a full sweat suit and a smile. He looks me up and down, curious and amused, but only when I am not looking at him. (The use of peripheral vision is indispensable in our work; one learns to be a periscope—to see but not be seen seeing.) He walks, sits on the floor, walks, sits on the floor. He folds his arms and crosses his legs, then repeats it all. He never speaks; has never, it is said, uttered a sound. He will not let me touch him. He finally lets me touch his hands. He is known for smearing the walls with his excrement (common asylum behavior which I haven't yet had the privilege of witnessing).

The first two sessions, with Baba and Little Joe, are

encouraging. When I see Lekbir for the first time, however, I am suddenly confused: he does not fit the other
two suspects' MO at all—it's apples and oranges.
Whereas it makes perfect sense to say that Baba and Little
Joe resemble each other in terms of their behavior—you
could say that they "have" the same condition—one
cannot at all say as much for Lekbir. Yes, he manifests
stereotypical gestures, but they are insignificant, unre-
markable ones; yes, he avoids eye contact, but in a way
that any normal shy person might (and the same goes
for his "air of aloneness"); he scratches himself, but
rarely breaks the skin, seems uninterested in what's happening around him . . . that is, until I suddenly sit down
on the floor and cross my legs exactly as he's done. Now
he's *very* interested.

During the twenty sessions of imitation, Baba will
demonstrate much greater interest in me than he ever
has in anyone; we communicate through our mutual
gestures and chicken-clucking mouth sounds. Lekbir imitates everything I do, absolutely everything, usually behind my back—I'll sit down and cross my legs, right leg
over left, with my hands in my lap, and he'll sit down on
the floor and do exactly the same thing, then I'll cross
my legs, left leg over right, and he'll immediately follow
suit. The staff teases me about turning a serious scientific research project into a game of Jacques-a-dit (the
French version of Simon Says). Little Joe, undoubtedly
the most hermetically sealed autistic person I've ever

worked with, toward the end of the twenty sessions will—O rapture!—wink at me exactly once.

The year and a half that I spent at Ventose taught me several important lessons. The least important is that one should never take people's good faith for granted. My presence in this old, somewhat hidden psychiatric department, though much appreciated by most, was also roundly resented by others (none of whom worked on our project); I was accused of slumming: "What's this American dude doing down here, snooping around and playing dress-up with our patients? He's grandstanding at their expense. Next thing you know, he's going to put them on television." The staff of interns who had seemed delighted at the idea of analyzing the videocassettes and marking the results on the behavioral grid sheets in the end did neither.

The most important thing I learned was that even in the profoundly autistic, age has less relevance to behavioral change than we tend to think. The phenomenon of reciprocal imitation on the one hand, and the successful building of affective relationships on the other, was neither easier nor more difficult to come by in these older people than they are in autistic children. This has since been demonstrated to me many times.

A third conclusion, the most puzzling one, has in fact only recently occurred to me; it arose in the course of my writing these pages. By the time I created my own institution in suburban Paris in 1997, among many other kinds of work I had been imitating autistic people on and off for over twenty-four years. For the last six years, I've had the pleasure of sharing the same kind of exceptional relationship that I had with Adam S. back in the early seventies in Detroit (and with others since then) with all our thirty-odd autistic-spectrum children, adolescents and young adults. According to the people I've been working with for more than a decade, my empathic gifts are richer than ever.

Imagine my surprise, then, when it dawned on me a few months ago that I haven't imitated an autistic person in at least five years.

What is empathy? *Blakiston's Medical Dictionary* (it happens to be sitting next to me, which is the only reason I keep referring to it) defines "empathy" as "[t]he vicarious experience of another person's situation and psychological state, which may facilitate intuitive understanding of that person's feelings, thoughts, and actions."

Is this vicarious experience something we cause—on purpose or by accident—or something that happens *to* us? Are we born with a predisposition to have it, or is it an acquired skill? Can human beings empathize with nonhumans? If so, which kinds? Animals? Plants? Paintings? Music? Wallpaper? When someone says, "I feel your pain," is it really *your* pain that he or she is feeling, or is it the person's own pain, which he or she assumes (on what grounds?) to be the equivalent, qualitatively and quantitatively, of yours? ("Your dog died? I know exactly how you feel—I got turned down for a supporting role on *The Sopranos* last week.") Can one empathize with another person's situation or psychological state, having never been in either exactly the same situation or exactly the same psychological state? How exactly the same do situations and psychological states have to be to qualify? Most pertinently put: *Can one empathize with another person's situation and psychological state while having no firsthand knowledge of what it's like to be that person?*

If we rely on certain psychoanalytic hypotheses about where the autistic state comes from (a psychological trauma early in life) and what it represents (a defense against what is thus perceived to be an intolerable world), then the possibility that a nonautistic person could claim firsthand knowledge of such a state seems dicey to me.

If, on the other hand, we hypothesize that the autistic state arises from a complex disharmony in the way the brain treats sensory information, a state which prevents the person from being able to adequately control or make sense of his or her immediate environment, then it would seem possible that by imitating an autistic person thoroughly, in detail and for long periods of time, we could obtain firsthand, *visceral* knowledge of the state in which that autistic person finds himself or herself.

Current research tends to favor the second hypothesis. In the absence of imitation, my empathy remains. Where does it come from? A year or so ago, on entering the institution early one afternoon, I came upon a certain Dirka, a young nonverbal Kurdish autistic woman, sitting on the couch in the lobby, surrounded by three distraught *éducatrices spécialisées* (special-ed people, female). Dirka was crying her eyes out, screaming. She'd been like this for an hour, I was told. Maybe she had a toothache—she'd been putting her fingers deep into her mouth all morning—but the Tylenol they'd given her hadn't helped at all. I stood there watching, as helpless as the rest. Then, for a reason that I will never understand, it became patently obvious to me what I had to do. I kneeled down in front of her, took her into my arms and hugged her while pushing with my two hands on a specific spot on the middle-right side of her back. Dirka stopped crying immediately. She put her arms around me. The three *éducatrices* filed out of the lobby, dabbing their eyes.

Where does this empathy come from, and how did it get there?

One explanation, a rather philosophical one, comes to mind. Having "been there, done that" for so long (it's true that, empirically speaking, I've probably had some kind of imitative truck with every different "type" of autistic person known), I can now simply let my body remember what it felt like to "be" each of them, and let a specific empathy build itself out of what my body remembers.

Here's a more intriguing idea: What if my years of intense imitating (my physical and mental investment in the act has always gone well beyond simple monkey-see, monkey-do) has enabled me to develop, from the outside in, my own forms of cross-modal sensory associations, associations that enable me to "feel, see, smell and hear" with my eyes what the autistic person I'm looking at feels, sees, smells or hears in his or her body?

The project at Ventose, in addition to everything else, left me bewildered about how we go about categorizing autistic people—or any other kind of people, for that matter—and how untrustworthy such enterprises can be.

The three men with whom I was to conduct my study, Baba, Little Joe and Lekbir, supposedly constituted a rigorously obtained homogeneous sample—they all checked out against the same long list of behavioral criteria—and yet in the end turned out to constitute a sample that was barely two-thirds homogeneous. How is this possible? What does this mean?

Psychiatry is a branch of medicine. Psychiatric diagnosis uses the medical diagnostic model. One may conceive of medical diagnostics as having four major components: (1) the symptoms; (2) the cause of these symptoms (etiology); (3) the name of the condition; and

(4) the treatment indicated. By symptoms we mean so-matic—bodily—anomalies. These might also be called atypical and harmful behaviors of the organism. By cause, or etiology, we mean the biological or genetic agent or agents whose presence in the body is responsi-ble for the existence of the observed symptoms (bacte-ria, viruses, toxins, mutations). Treatment means the administration of medicinal agents—chemical or nat-ural—physical interventions (e.g., surgery) and/or non-medicinal somatic interventions (e.g., physiotherapy) whose function is to annul the symptoms.

We might imagine a chart with four columns on it: Symptoms, Diagnosis, Etiology, Treatment. A person goes to see a doctor. He is coughing and he is running a fever. Using a stethoscope, the doctor ascertains that there is also fluid and congestion in the patient's lungs. She marks these symptoms in the Symptoms column of the chart. The doctor then consults her diagnostic manual, in which she finds that fever + coughing + congestion and fluid in the lungs = bacterial pneumonia. The doctor marks "bacterial pneumonia" in the Diagnosis column. Symptoms play a definitive role in determining diagno-sis. Thus armed with a diagnosis, the doctor now con-sults her pathology manual to see what causes bacterial pneumonia. In the Etiology column she writes "staphy-lococcus infection." Diagnosis plays a definitive role in determining etiology. Anxious to counteract the disease, the doctor looks in her clinical practice book and learns that the treatment of choice for bacterial pneumonia is penicillin (or a similar antibiotic). She writes "penicillin" in the Treatment column of the chart. Etiology plays a definitive role in determining treatment. Unfortunately, a week later the patient calls and informs the doctor that all the symptoms are still present. This being the case, the doctor calls into question her diagnosis—her idea of what is wrong with the patient—maybe it's a huge cold, maybe viral pneumonia. . . . Treatment plays a definitive role in determining the ultimate diagnosis.

The parents of a young child notice that he's behaving strangely: he doesn't look at his mother when she nurses him; he seems distant. They take him to see a child psychiatrist. The psychiatrist asks lots of questions, looks over the child's medical history, spends some time alone with the child, observes certain oddities in his behavior. The doctor writes these things, and the others he's been told about, in the Symptoms column. He looks in the diagnostic manual and realizes that the child demonstrates many of the symptoms associated with autism (or the autistic spectrum). He writes "autism" in the Diagnosis column.

What will the psychiatrist write in the two columns still left empty: Etiology and Treatment?

Much research has been done concerning the etiology of autism. Hypotheses abound. Some people still believe that bad parenting in the first months of life causes autism. Some believe that multiple vaccination shots containing mercury—which may stagnate for decades in the blood, thus instigating mercury poisoning—is responsible. Some people suspect that allergies to certain foods—wheat gluten, for example—play a role in the cause of autism. Others blame innate or acquired sensory anomalies—hearing that's too sensitive or not sensitive enough, or, as mentioned earlier, cross-modal sensory associations (see page 60). Current genetic research is beginning to provide clues, such as the systematic chromosomal alignment of amino acids in a certain order found in some autistic subjects.

There are people who satisfy the diagnostic criteria for autism and in whose brains we find lesions. Might we thus be justified in holding these lesions responsible for the autistic symptoms we observe, or should we assume that they have nothing to do with them? Might we hold them responsible for some of the symptoms and not others? Which ones? How do we explain the fact that other diagnostically autistic people do not have any brain lesions at all? Are we to presume that the people who have brain lesions are the "real" autistics, because the presumed source of their condition is observable, as are bacteria and viruses in other diseases—or, on the contrary, are they "false" autistics, since "presence of cerebral anomalies" does not figure among today's official diagnostic criteria?

Margaret Bauman, the Boston neurologist mentioned earlier, has discovered that many autistic brains contain abnormally small, abnormally numerous neurons in the hippocampal complex, which would indicate a finite period of accelerated brain growth early in life.* Though such findings are not mentioned in any existing diagnostic assessment resource, might they someday become the primary criterion for autism?

The true cause of autism thus remaining a mystery, and no sure treatments—pharmacological, psychological, nutritional, environmental—having been found as of this writing, the medical model columns headed Etiology and Treatment are still empty. As long as this situation endures, the diagnostic label of autism will serve as just that, a label, and not much else. Labels can be useful, though. They may be employed as research tools; under most circumstances, they help us in obtaining reliable, relatively homogeneous samples (my project with Lekbir, Baba and Little Joe notwithstanding), and in the United States they are necessary in order to secure the therapeutic and educational services the person is entitled to by law.

In our work as psychotherapists we often talk about "treating the person" as opposed to "treating the illness."

---

* M. Bauman, *The Neurology of Autism,* in online journal published by the Interdisciplinary Council on Developmental and Learning Disorders, January 2002.

Autism is widely recognized today as an innate disorder and not as a "mental illness." An innate disorder is something one is born with; an illness is something one "catches." As a rule one does not catch autism, though several of the hypotheses mentioned above concerning its cause—food allergies, for example—would, if proven true, put the lie to this statement.

I am often under the impression that people diagnosed as autistic tend to differ from one another more than do the people diagnosed with certain other innate disorders, such as Down syndrome or Rett's Disorder.* Because of the wide range of autistic profiles and personalities, when conferring with colleagues we in the business tend to describe our clients in terms of other clients: *You remember Tim? Right. Well, the kid I'm sending over is just like Tim, only his speech is like a cross between Amanda's and Harvey's, and his stereotypy is the same as Bill. . . . You know how Bill flaps his hands? Exactly like Bill, only with his arms rigid like Dorothy and rocking like Irv. Not Big Irv, Little Irv. The one who reminds us of Steve.*

How are the lines drawn? Simply put, autism, properly speaking, always distinguishes itself by the presence of that "glass wall"—the "air of aloneness when one is

---

* A congenital neurodegenerative condition occurring only in females, some of whose symptoms—language deficit, stereotypical hand movements and loping gait—resemble those of autism.

not alone"—that Leo Kanner described. (At first he thought these children were deaf. They're not.)

I sometimes think that the easiest way to distinguish a true autistic person from the others is to see if they turn around when you call.

Somatic maladies are consistent; they almost always behave predictably, in accordance with their diagnostic names. Autism does not. Very few autistic people *never* turn around when you call them; sometimes they do. Various hypotheses concerning the peculiar, fluctuating sensory states of the autistic—hearing, for example— could explain this phenomenon. Or one could imagine that a particular psychological state—overwhelming distraction or intense concentration on something that we don't see (say, a spot on the ceiling)—may be at work in the glass-wall effect. Even in the cases where an autistic child makes great progress and most of his symptoms all but disappear, there almost always remains this trace, this air, this invisible cloud of distance, this ever so slightly noticeable air of aloneness that sets these people apart from us normopaths.

In the meantime, it is important not to confuse this distinguishingly autistic trait with certain behaviors we notice in normal people—normally melancholy people, for example, who feel "alone in a crowd" and let it show. The neighbor's teenage son, plugged into his Walkman twenty-four hours a day, who never comes out of his room. Your mother-in-law, who has never once said a word when she comes over for dinner. The mailman, who has never in the thirteen years you've been living in your house looked you in the eye. And you yourself, who can't help but go back into the kitchen fifteen times to make absolutely sure that you shut the water off before going out to get the paper. Stop flattering yourselves. You are not autistic. The *autistic* are autistic.

As chickenpox does not change into mumps, so schizophrenia does not evolve into manic depression. Short of being declared cured, or of being rediagnosed by someone new, one usually carries one's psychiatric diagnosis for life—once autistic, always autistic—even if certain adjectives may be added on to insinuate levels of severity. Nor does the progress that certain of our young customers make while in our care help us much as we wade around in the diagnostic mire. The clearly diagnosable autistic person who previously would sit on a chair only if it was yellow and who never came out of his alcove in the hall where he sat rocking and who now sits in chairs of all colors and seems to be delighted to be with other people—were we to meet him today for the first time, it is possible that we would not issue a diagnosis of autism. Yet if this were true, which diagnosis would be correct? The one originally issued five years ago, or the one issued today by someone meeting the person for the first time?

The term Autistic Spectrum Disorder, which as noted earlier has come into wide use, at least in North America, is a handy one. Deliberately broad in scope, it allows those benefiting from it to qualify for care and educational programs—programs mandated by state or federal law, as mentioned—yet does not reduce the recipient of the diagnosis to a rigid, standard, one-definition-fits-all stereotype. ("That's an autistic child? Why, he doesn't look anything like the one I saw in the TV movie last night on Lifetime!") A virtue of the term Autistic Spectrum Disorder is that it intrinsically implies the diversity of the people it applies to. Quality caregivers always customize their care plans according to the specificities of the individual; it simply makes no sense to use the same techniques in the same way with everybody. This applies not only to the question of *which* technique is suitable but also to *how* the technique should be utilized. A minimum of empathy helps us to know when to be firm, silly, distant, cajoling, harsh, mushy, frightening or attractive in the eyes of the young client sitting in front of us (or swinging from the chandelier overhead). Our choice of which attitude to "wear" will dictate how efficient or inefficient the chosen technique will be.

Autism is not only not a household word in France; when it is used, it is often used incorrectly. Despite the obvious particulars that distinguish most *psychotiques* from most *autistes*—the capacity to build relationships (albeit sometimes perverted or unhealthy ones), language skills, IQ levels (varying widely from case to case), the presence of hallucinations, etc.—opportunities to explain in detail what distinguishes one term from another are rare. Nor is the term Autistic Spectrum Disorder widely used; in fact, it's possible that it never will be: *le Spectre Autistique* (the official translation) not only means the Autistic Spectrum; it also means the Autistic Ghost. For the time being, the French today, professionals included, will probably just continue to use the word *autiste* to describe everything from classical Kanner autism to pervasive developmental disorders, mental retardation and, yes, your silent mother-in-law.

4

IMPOSTERS

I remember the television we had when I was five. It was a brownish-beige piece of self-contained furniture, with a screen more round than square on which I watched *The Mickey Mouse Club* every weekday afternoon. What I remember most about watching *The Mickey Mouse Club* every weekday afternoon was how I had to comb my hair before I sat down; my hair had to be combed very carefully—I had a "Princeton" haircut, and the little snatch of long hair in front had to be perfectly shaped so as to glide gracefully backward in a sculpted wave that disappeared gradually into the buzz cut field behind. It took hours. What also took hours was getting dressed up in the starched white shirt, the black Elvis pants, and the loafers with no stitching that I always wore while watching *The Mickey Mouse Club*. Thus

111

dressed and groomed, I could confidently sit myself down in the nubby brown easy chair and wait, trembling, for Annette to walk onto the screen. When Annette walked onto the screen, I'd sit up little-soldier straight and flash her my most sensitive smile.

When Annette walked onto the screen, she always looked at me first. She had to be looking at me; I was the only one there.

I realized, of course, that certain things about *The Mickey Mouse Club* escaped logical reason (I was only five, but I wasn't stupid): The Mouseketeers, for example—the ten or so Mouseketeers—I knew that they couldn't all be inside the television. . . . There wasn't enough room! (Unless, of course, the Mouseketeers were really only five inches tall, a hypothesis as difficult to swallow as the hypothesis that they were really in black and white.)

What was certain is that Annette existed—I was in love with her, she had to—and if someone exists, he or she has to be somewhere. But if the real Annette, who in all probability was *Homo sapiens*–life-size, couldn't possibly fit into the television, who was that on the screen? It still had to be Annette!

There was only one explanation possible: Annette existed somewhere (I was in love with her, she had to), and there was only one of her (same reasoning). The Annette who looked at me and whom I saw inside the television had to be the one and only Annette; just not the same one.

This kind of reasoning seems paradoxical—how can "the one and only Annette" not be "the same one"?

I am sitting at my computer keyboard, typing this sentence. It is 1:47 P.M. in Paris. In my wallet in my pocket is my New York driver's license with a photograph of me on it. Am I not the same person as the person in the photograph? Of course not: I am a Howard Buten who is typing this sentence; the other person is a Howard Buten who is in a photograph on a driver's license. We are not the same size, we have different amounts of hair (what a difference four years make!) and we are doing different things. Yet according to the phone book, birth registry and (the most exhaustive source, I bet) the list of existing e-mail addresses, there exists only one Howard Buten. Still, I'm telling you, it's not the same one.

I am not the only person who thinks this way. Martin does too. Let me introduce you to him. . . .

I am stretched out on a picnic table by a bush in the courtyard of our clinic after lunch. Lunch was a grand event today. Emotions were high. (I'm thinking Mount Vesuvius, or was that Hurricane Ethel?) For a moment I thought it was snowing, but it was only the *macédoine de legumes,* falling like green hail on the heads of all twenty-two clients and half as many caregivers. I'm sunning myself on the picnic table. I'm falling asleep . . . disappearing into the Special Ed Void . . . Psychology Middle Earth. . . . Suddenly the bush begins to speak.

"Look, you can leave the kids alone for the five minutes it'll take you to pick Jean-Claude up at his house, okay?"

"What? Speak up. I can't hear you."

"What are you, deaf? Your telephone portable is really—"

"Where did you park the car? The Peugeot or the Citroen? Anyway, we can walk to the cinema!"

"Are you crazy? For once I get a good spot, and you—"

We are not budgeted for talking bushes. I deduce that something less vegetal is at work.

"Martin? Is that you behind the bush?"

"Okay, Martin! You're going to be punished! You're going to stay home with Jean and I don't want to hear another word—"

"Martin . . ."

"I'm in my world."

Martin goes into his world. Martin's world is not a matter of delirium—he never confuses it with the real world, nor is it hallucinatory—hallucinations are the province of schizophrenia, not autism. Schizophrenics cannot stop their hallucinations, whereas Martin comes back easily from his world if you ask him to. Though sometimes you have to ask a few times.

Martin is in his world right now. . . .

"We can't with this hitting! Uh, stop making noise! We can't with this hitting! Say what? Say what? Say what? He doesn't know how to listen! We can't with . . . **WHAT IF I HOLD HIM?** . . . He wants the blurry TV. Honestly I'm telling you, I . . . Who knows why? **OKAY, MARTIN, YOU'RE GONNA TALK INTO THE TAPE RECORDER, BUT YOU WON'T BE ABLE TO KEEP IT! I WANT TO GO TO VILLE D'AVRAY! YOU WON'T BE ABLE TO KEEP IT! I WANT THE BLURRY TV! THIS ONE'S ON THE BLINK DOMMAGE! I DON'T WANT TO BE DISAPPOINTED. WELL, YOU'RE GOING TO BE DISAPPOINTED! YOU'RE GOING . . . YOU'RE GOING TO BE VERY DISAPPOINTED!** What'll you do if I stop the wheels? **YOU'LL GET SLAPPED! WORK IT OUT WITH YOUR MOTHER!** When are we going to sit down to dinner? Are there crêpes? **SIT DOWN? YOU BROKE THE CHAIR! NOW YOU'RE GOING TO HAVE TO FIX IT! YES, YOU CAN. YOU KNOW YOU CAN!** Come over here and help me. . . . David's going to run out, and he can have one of the baguettes. . . . He'll be number 'one' and you number 'two' . . . and 'three,' so we'll have numbers here. . . . We should have figures on TV! Look,

I want him to open . . . *YOU CUT THAT OUT RIGHT NOW, OR I'M CALLING YOUR MOTHER!"*

As we have noted earlier, the category high-functioning autism pertains to autistic people who, despite their deficiencies in communicating, in relating, in affect and in showing interest in what goes on around them, can more or less function on their own in society (note that the "more or less" is important). Some possess a special gift or talent worthy of genius. In French this kind of person is referred to as an *autiste à capacité spéciale,* an autistic with a special talent.

Martin imitates people. He has imitated people since he was three (he's fifteen now). He reproduces people's voices: their speech patterns, their tones of voice, their vocabularies—the people who work at the clinic, his parents, movie stars, me. He imitates the screams and vocalizations of the other young people at the clinic so well that if we don't see with our own eyes who's vocalizing, we can never be sure whether it's them or Martin, the Great Imposter. This can be very troubling. He can reproduce the entire sound track of certain films—dialogue, music and sound effects. He can also do it backward if you like, or in slow motion. (Paradoxically, when he speaks as himself, his voice is flat, without nuance or modulation, a singsong binary cadence that never varies.) At the clinic Martin's supernatural talents never cease to amaze us, but at home he is intolerable.

In his bedroom Martin obsesses on his tape recorder; he plasters his ear against the speaker and goes into ecstasy. He runs out in the hallway, runs back in his room, runs out in the hallway. He rewinds and replays and rewinds, pushing down the buttons in such a way as to make the tape play backward at triple speed for hours and hours and hours. "It sounds like an elf," he explains. And Martin talks to himself out loud at home, repeating the same things again and again: "I want Françoise! I want Françoise! I want Françoise!" (Françoise is a young aide who rode in the school bus with him last year.) "Want the blurry TV! Want *La Famille Addams*!" and he's all over his mother, then he's all over his father, pulling on their sleeves. "Want to live in Maurice's house!" (an intern from two years ago). "I'm going to rip my clothes apart! I can't stop myself!" This is Martin in his world, where an endless litany of multiple voices on a high-speed track drown out everything anyone might say in an effort to burst the bubble. Into the kitchen, back to his room, past his little brother and sister, across through the den.

At the clinic he throws things—out the window, through the mail slot, down the toilet, out the door. Papers, shoes, cups, magazines, pencils, underpants, string. *I can't stop myself! I can't! I can't!* He wants to see where things go, he says: balloons let go, papers that blow, water down the drain, clouds in the sky. Where does it go next? "Out the window, Martin." And after the window? "The roof, Martin." And after the roof? "The sky, Martin." And after the sky? "Heaven, Martin." And after Heaven? "God, Martin." And after God? "County Mental Health, Martin." And after County Mental Health? "There's nothing after County Mental Health, Martin." And Martin lies. He confesses to having tossed the shoe we can't find over the fence into the neighbor's yard and that we have to find it and that he couldn't stop himself. (We find it ten minutes later, behind the door.) Martin rips his clothes apart. He dismantles electronic equipment. He admonishes us ceaselessly about a certain Nicolas Bouvier (apparently the name of a puppet Martin uses to masturbate with, or the name of a boy he knew at day camp, or hypothetically both and probably neither). Martin drools on windowpanes. "To imitate Nicolas Bouvier," he says. (Which?) He monopolizes both his parents, crying out in nonstop anguish, "Something's wrong inside me!" (true? false?) all night long.

What theoretical base can a psychologist rely on to understand why Martin behaves as he does? What techniques can help us sort out his brilliant word salad, the extreme emotions it puts him through, the meaning of it all?

There are distinctions between the school of Gestalt psychology founded by Max Wertheimer, Wolfgang Köhler and Kurt Koffka in Germany in the 1920s and 1930s, and the school of Gestalt psychotherapy founded by Fritz Perls in California in the 1960s.

Wertheimer, Köhler and Koffka were interested in how human beings—their brains, their minds—treat sensory perception. How do we *cognate*—"make of it in our minds"—all that we see, hear, touch, smell? Certain scientific experiments of the time suggested that humans tend to perceive things as wholes rather than as a series of parts. For example, a vertical bar of light that falls on its side in rapid, discrete increments is perceived as falling in one continual, unbroken movement.

A "gestalt" is defined as a whole, the nature of which is unchanged by changes in its parts. When we look at a square, for example, we recognize it as a square. Even if there is a little chunk missing from one of its sides, or if there are a few tiny chunks missing here and there, or if it's polka-dotted or striped, big or small, turned this way or that, to our perceptive eye it's still a square—it retains its squareness, its square gestalt.

Wertheimer, Köhler and Koffka were not therapists. They were not particularly interested in studying emotional states in people. Their interest was in understanding how human minds alter what their five senses perceive. They were also philosophers—that people tend to perceive fragmented shapes as being whole (remember the blinking bar of light and the unfinished squares) seemed to them to say something important about the nature of all humanity. But Perls borrowed the perceptual concept of gestalt and applied it to the problems of emotional life. According to Perls, we tend to experience our lives—interpersonal relationships, conscious or unconscious memories, emotional situations (falling in love, getting bawled out)—as emotional gestalts. These gestalts may be "open" or "closed." If someone feels bad, ill at ease or sorrowful, it's likely that somewhere in his or her life there's a relationship, memory or situation that is experienced as being "unclosed"—an open gestalt that needs closure.

Perls believed that these open gestalts have to be experienced as closed—emotionally, empirically, here and now, through live action—for the person to feel better and be able to get on with his or her life. Talking about it does not suffice. (For Freud, on the other hand, this task is accomplished solely by talking in the psychoanalytic setting. This leads to transference—the projecting of the problems one has or had with his or her parents onto the psychoanalyst himself, which allows the patient to then resolve them with the psychoanalyst. This is not a behavioral process; it is a psychic one: it happens only in the mind and, up until the end, without your knowing it.)

Because for Perls the unfinished situation has to be experienced, albeit symbolically, for the person to feel the closure of the open gestalt, Perls invented a panoply of "games" to be played (out) during therapy sessions—

role-playing alone or with others, two-chair exercises, anger-venting pillow punching—which are guided by the therapist, often, but not always, in a group situation.

I ask Martin to sit in one of the two chairs I've placed face-to-face in the room. I seat myself in a third chair, at a right angle a yard away.

"Look at the chair in front of you, Martin. Using your brain images (Martin's always talking about his 'brain images'), imagine that Martin is sitting there in front of you. Martin-2. You're Martin-1. Sitting in front of you is Martin-2."

"It's not the same one."

"We'll see about that. . . ."

"Want to go back to being the 'MartinWhoCame-Before.'"

"Good idea. Look at Martin-2, Martin, sitting in front of you. He'll be the MartinWhoCameBefore."

(Huge smile, hand flapping, five seconds of imitating a blurry TV . . .)

"It's him!"

"It is. Say something to him."

(In his father's voice) "No, no, no . . . What do you think you're . . . Oh, great, you broke the tape recorder again. . . ."

"No. I want Martin-1 to talk to the MartinWho-CameBefore."

"It won't be the same one."

"Whatever . . ."

"There's Martin-1 and Martin-2."

"Ask Martin-2 if he wants to still be autistic."

"I'm scared to stop being autistic."

"Ask Martin-2."

"I'm scared."

"How do you know?"

"You told me."

It's true. Some time ago I offered the hypothesis that Martin might be frightened by the idea of not being autistic anymore, and that this might explain some of his anxiety, his obsessions. He hadn't, thus far, given me his opinion.

"Martin. Ask Martin-2."

Martin looks at the other chair. "You're afraid to not still be autistic."

"Now, go sit in the other chair. (He does.) Good. Now, Martin-2, answer Martin-1."

(In my voice) "Look, buddy, just deal with it!"

"Martin-2, MartinWhoCameBefore, I'd like you to answer Martin-1's question."

The notion of gestalt—of living the events of daily life as being "open" or "closed," "finished" or "unfinished"— seems pertinent to what I imagine to be the autistic experience, in big ways and small.

Repetitive gestures—rocking, hand flapping, finger gazing—act not only as a form of self-hypnosis but also as a kind of unending physical quest toward the finishing of something that is never finished. Their analgesic effect must be perpetually renewed; every time autistics finish, they must start over again. No matter how many hours they may spend rocking back and forth in the corner of the room, the sensory thirst of the autistic is never quenched for long; the proprioceptive gestalt no sooner closes than it opens again.

One often observes certain autistic people who spin themselves as they walk along—one full turn to the right in mid-trajectory for no apparent reason, then one full turn to the left in the same spot on the way back. They seem to be "winding" themselves in one direction, then "unwinding" themselves in the other—opening the lid of some internal jar, then closing it again—starting something for no reason other than to have something left to finish, finishing it for no reason other than to have something to start. It's very satisfying.

Closing all the windows; turning all the bottles so that the labels face the same way; touching every object in the room with your index finger and then doing it again in the same order; swiveling the armchair so it faces the wall and not tolerating its being swiveled back by someone else . . . one can see how opening and closing the tiny gestalts of daily life allow autistic people to feel that they can control their environment, that they

can "do" things, *these* things—do them all day long
without ever being threatened, as we are, by the infinitely more abstract, more important (to us, anyway)
and infinitely more dangerous things that are, no matter
how you look at it, much harder to ever "feel finished"
about: work, love, ambition, religion, art, success,
death. . . .

Martin is preoccupied by his voice; he's anxious for it to
change, to get deeper. He keeps asking when this will
happen; he asks fifty times a day. He rips up his clothes
less now; he imitates the blurry TV less; he throws his
clothes out the window less; he's less obsessed by tape
recorders; he's more with us when he's with us.

This is how Martin handles growing up: he tells us
he's scared of becoming an adult; he tells us he's anxious
to become an adult; he tells us he's impatient to become
an adult; he tells us he's worried about becoming an
adult. He says he's afraid of losing the MartinWho-
CameBefore—of having to leave behind the Martin who
was in his world all the time. He wants to know what
the MartinWhoComesAfter will be like, and when he'll
come. It won't be the same one, he says.

Martin wonders about "the same one." In the video
room at the clinic, a group is viewing a tape made two
years ago. Martin is watching, seated on a brown chair.
In the video we see Martin and the others in the video

room at the clinic two years ago. The brown chair appears on the screen. Martin watches the screen—he's sitting on the brown chair, watching the screen.

"That's this chair!" he says, looking earnestly at me.

"Yes, Martin, it is."

His face empties itself of all emotion, the sign that he's thinking.

"It's not the same one."

I note in my pad to look up what "virtual" really means.

Time marches on. Martin tells us he wants to attend a normal school. What serendipity—we recently got the ball rolling on a project to create an integrated classroom in the *collège* (the French for junior high school) around the corner. When I tell this to Martin, he starts to cry. "I want to stay autistic!" His lips tremble, the tears flow. At the same time, I notice a trace of a smile appearing at the corners of his mouth—a trace of a trace of a smile. It's Martin all over; the role-playing, the actor. I tell him I understand. I explain that if he wants to go to a normal school, he will in fact have to become more normal and, alas, less autistic. I allow as how in his shoes I'd be scared too, and that no matter what, I will always be there for him.

I take out a piece of paper and divide it into two columns, headed NORMAL CHILD and AUTISTIC CHILD. In the first column I write a list of characteristics that describe a normal child, and in the second I

write a list of characteristics that describe Martin. I read
it out loud. Martin cries harder.

"It will always be you who decides, Martin. Always.
Nothing is written in stone; you can change your mind
whenever you like. You can always go back to being
autistic." He looks me straight in the eye. His tears dry
a little. He takes my hand, leans toward me. "Now, it
would be convenient for me if you managed to become
a little more normal. That way you could participate
more with other human beings—your parents, for example, or your brother, or your sister, or me. But the
choice is yours. It will always be you who decides."

He starts trembling again.

"I want to be autistic."

"Okay, Martin. Fine. If that's—"

"I want to be normal."

"What? Oh. Well, okay, then—"

"What's 'written in stone'?"

Self-injurious behavior is common in the autistic. They
bite their hands, their wrists; they hit their heads against
the wall; they pound their heads with their hands,
screaming; they tear their skin off, shred by shred; they
push their fingers in their eyes up to the knuckle; sometimes they use objects to hurt themselves, and sometimes
they use people. What they rarely do, though, is commit
suicide.

We assume it's about frustration—the inability to express themselves otherwise. We assume it's about feeling themselves—the limits of their bodies, the frontier between what's them and what's not them. We wonder if this sensation searching is due to an overdose of the endogenous opiate pentapeptides in the brain, like the endorphins we've mentioned earlier.

Little by little Martin begins to destroy himself. He loses control, goes off the deep end. He comes to us screaming—eyes closed, face twisted. "There's something's that's wrong with me! There's something that's wrong with me!" Some think: Martin, Oscar nominee for Best Actor in a Clinical Setting, is just doing his thing; he wants attention. When asked what it is that's wrong, he screams that he doesn't know. He starts breaking things: plates and glasses at lunch, toys and windows at recess. And then himself. "I want to go back to the Martin-WhoCameBefore!" he screams, throwing himself into the wall.

The decision to hospitalize Martin is hard to make. He asks for it himself, begs for it. He wants to be given medication; he wants to be examined by doctors; he wants to spend all day in pajamas. We finally admit him to a psychiatric hospital. The next morning he wants out. Back home again, he takes to assembling chairs into walls that he erects between himself and the objects that he can't keep himself from destroying: clocks, televisions, mirrors. He howls like a wolf for hours on end. I can't stop myself! Help me! *Help Me!* He never sleeps. He slaps his mother.

His psychological disarray is dramatic, his pain heartbreaking. And yet, again, at the corners of his mouth, twisted in true anguish, we seem to perceive the smallest trace of a smile, drowning as it is in Martin's bitter, very real tears. Is this the work of a charlatan, an imposter? The Great Tragedian, his play himself: the extravagance of the artistic autistic? On this the staff is divided. The debate rages.

Decidedly, there's something's wrong.

There was a famous quote, oft repeated in the sixties, recounted by E. M. Forster in *Aspects of the Novel*: "I'll know what I think when I see what I say."

On the subway I start writing ideas down in random order, then I start moving them around. The next morning I submit my patchwork hypotheses to the staff.

SCHEMATIC RECENT
REFLECTIONS ON MARTIN

Martin's recent behavior reflects a state of true fear: the fear of a psychological void. This void has been created by the absence of affective object relations that otherwise give meaning to life: Love, Friendship, Caring, Sharing, Pride, Shame, Generosity, Empathy. The incapacity to feel these things is in the nature of autism. Up until now Martin has been using classical autistic defenses to fend off this non-autistic void—gestural stereotypy, vocal stereotypy, isolation.

But for some time now we've observed a clear drop in Martin's stereotypical behaviors and isolation. His autistic defense system, his autism itself, seems to be disappearing.

The anxiety Martin is experiencing is, by definition, nonautistic. (There's nothing autistic in experiencing real anxiety because of a real void.) Yet what means of defense are now left him to combat the real anxiety produced by the void?

Answer: Martin, brilliant as always, has found a way to use anxiety itself as a defense against anxiety: he "plays" it. As soon as he feels anxiety coming on, he starts "acting" anxious—repeating sobs and screams by rote, like lines from a play. Martin's anxiety is at once both real and pretend.

(Note: I often think about the passage in *The Catcher in the Rye* in which Holden Caulfield gets punched in the stomach by a thug bellboy in the hotel hallway. Bent over in pain, he stumbles back into his room. As he passes the open doorway leading to the bathroom, he suddenly sees himself in the bathroom mirror, face twisted in pain. Watching himself, he begins to act, twisting his face even more, hamming it up—playing his own role in a film of himself.)

If it's true that Martin's old defense system is disappearing, it must be because the autistic void is somehow getting filled. We already see signs of Friendship, Generosity, Pride. This is progress.

Our strategy must be to help Martin rid himself of the new defense system, and at the same time help him fill the void.

What to do? First we should establish a generalized attitude toward Martin's theatrical defenses (when theatrical): make them disappear by depriving them of all reactions that acknowledge their existence. At the same time we must teach Martin the things that give meaning to life . . . by talking about them, and above all through our own example.

H. B., March 3 (odd-numbered day)

Question: How can one demonstrate what makes life worth living to an autistic person when what makes life worth living is affective relationships, which by definition the autistic person, being autistic, can't have?

Answer: Fake him out.

*   *   *

The superego is a Freudian psychic agency. Freudian psychic agencies are not things; they do not show up on X rays or MRIs. Psychic agencies are collections of psychic functions—they are what they do, like gravity. (One cannot see gravity. It has no material consistency, neither atoms nor waves; it exists only through its effects.) We observe a person's behavior—his or her emotional states and way of being under certain circumstances—and we try to describe the mechanisms behind it. Freud invented his psychic agencies—ego, id, superego—in his structural theory to explain, in part, the whys and wherefores of human behavior in the same way that Isaac Newton invented gravity to explain why things fall. When the theory of gravitation is no longer the most efficient way to explain why things fall, there will be no such thing as gravity and we'll have to find another concept to take its place. Some people believe that the Freudian psychoanalytical structural theory is already no longer the most efficient way to explain the whys and wherefores of human behavior.

The superego is the conscience of the unconscious. It tells us what's right to think and do and what's wrong. It is, in a way, our parents within us who survey and discipline. Shame and pride, avarice and generosity, ambition and humility are effects of the superego.

The Freudian superego is part of the unconscious; we don't feel it at work.

Martin imitates his parents. We hear him doing it so often at the clinic that when we find ourselves with his real parents, we are always a little confused. The content of Martin's parental imitation consists mostly of scolding. Martin speaks in the voices of dozens of different people, some who are recognizable and some who aren't. None of these voices ever has anything good to say about him.

According to Freud, the superego evolves through the process of introjection and identification. *Introjection* is a sort of psychological absorption of someone or something into our psyches. This process enables us to keep a representation, albeit an unconscious one, of the person or thing in our mind. *Identification* is the unconscious recognition in oneself of the person or thing introjected. To repeat: all of this is unconscious; it is not a matter of simple memories, but rather of memories we no longer remember but are nonetheless still there.

Martin does not feel pride or shame, or stinginess or generosity, or ambition or humility, all of which are products of the superego. This notwithstanding, he speaks to himself in his parents' voices, saying things they would say, bawling him out. He does this consciously.

One gets the feeling that Martin's superego is out there somewhere, walking around without him. How can we get it to go inside? If it doesn't, how is Martin ever to know pride, generosity, sanctions—all the qualities necessary to becoming a social being and without which life loses its meaning? Martin has already told us that he doesn't want to be autistic anymore.

Where can we find the Introjector of Martin's psyche?

An important experiment took place in the 1980s.* One-on-one, researchers instructed participants to adjust their facial features in certain ways ("Move the left corner of your mouth upward; bring the outside edge of your eyebrow down a half inch . . .") such that by the end of the adjustments, the participant could not know what his or her face looked like. At this point the participant was asked what kind of emotion, if any, he or she felt. Systematically, the subjects whose faces formed smiles said they felt happy, the subjects whose faces formed frowns said they felt unhappy and those whose faces had a perplexed look felt perplexed. What's more, the physiological markers of emotion—blood pressure, temperature, neurological activity by zone—also corresponded with the artificially created facial expression.

Until this time psychologists had assumed that a person's psychological state determined his or her behavior. This study demonstrated that the opposite can also be true.

What if the process of introjection—the unconscious psychological absorption of something or someone

---

* P. Ekman, R. W. Levenson, W. V. Friesen, "Autonomic Nervous System Activity Distinguishes among Emotions," *Science,* vol. 221 (1983), pp. 1208–10.

outside oneself into one's psyche—could be brought about through conscious, deliberate behavior?

Martin is happy that we're going to start doing theater again. We started this activity in 1998, a year after the center opened. We'd done it for two years, then stopped three years ago. Back then each session started with Martin's dictating the titles of the "plays" he wished to perform in. (Among the most noteworthy were *Martin Makes Doo-Doo in His Pants While Taking the Elevator*; *Howard Operates on Martin Because He Threw His Shoe into the Neighbor's Yard* and the ever popular *Robocop Falls Asleep in the Blurry TV.*) I made the posters.

This year, however, we're going to do things a little differently. There will be no more posters, and the plays will have no titles.

"Martin, we're going to work on the idea of consolation now."

"There's no more posters because why?"

"We're going to work on consolation."

"Okay, Martin, you can have some consolation, but if you break it, too bad for you!"

"When someone is sad or upset, say, and you try to be nice to this person so that they won't be sad or upset anymore, this is called consolation."

"Just deal with it, Buddy!"

134

"Take your mom, for example. . . ."

"Martin, your mom is really angry! Isn't that right, dear? That's right. I'm really angry!"

"Martin . . ."

"What?"

"Do you love your mom?"

"Yes."

"You know, sometimes she worries. . . ."

"I want the blurry TV. . . . Blurry TV? *No way!*"

"She's worried about you, Martin."

"I'm very worried, Dr. Buten. He ripped up his clothes again. . . ."

"Then if you love her, you should console her."

I demonstrate to Martin what a worried person looks like. I act it out. It's theater. I ask him to do like me. Martin acts out what a worried person looks like. Immediately I run over and take him in my arms. We repeat the scene. I congratulate him on his acting. Now we reverse the roles: I play Martin's mother, who is very worried because Martin has been breaking things at home. Mechanically, Martin takes me in his arms. We redo the scene; same result. "Do it for real!" I say. "Pretend that it's real!" I'm thinking about those researchers pointing to ligaments in people's faces.

Martin follows me up the stairs.

"You seem mad!" he says.

I nod. "See, Martin? You're making progress already."

"Why do you say that?"

"You recognize anger. You didn't before."

"You're mad because why?"

"You know why."

"I apologize!"

"Too late."

"I APOLOGIZE!"

"Do you know why I said that you're already making progress?"

"No."

"Because you understood that I'm mad. . . . Well, that I'm at least pretending to be mad . . ."

"It's just for fun."

". . . and that means that you're starting to feel in yourself what other people are feeling."

"No . . ."

"That's called 'empathy.' . . ."

"I'm going to break it."

". . . other people's feelings."

"They're not the same ones."

"If you only knew the half of it . . ."

Three months later Martin's mother calls me, very emotional. The previous evening he had been very late getting home from the clinic. When he came in the door, his mother said, "Martin! Thank goodness you're here!

I was worried sick!" And, according to her, Martin answered, "Don't worry, Mom. I'm here now."

For the first time in his life, Martin had consoled someone.

According to most authors, the lack of empathy is a formal criterion of autism. (This is distinguished from what is called the Theory of Mind,* another formal criterion of autism according to some. The Theory of Mind describes the ability to understand what other people are thinking, something else that autistic people can't do.) Autistic people often react inappropriately to their fellow autistics' emotional states. The sorrowful moaning of one can set off cascades of laughter in another, and vice versa.

Certain studies suggest that the autistic brain may treat visual information in such a way as to make it impossible for the autistic person to "read" other people's facial expressions, to discern their emotions. It's hard to empathize with someone if you can't tell by looking whether he's happy or sad.

The diagnostic criterion "flat affect" notwithstanding,

* S. Baren-Cohen, *Theory of Mind and Autism: A Fifteen-Year Review,* in eds. Baren-Cohen, H. Tager-Flusberg, and D. J. Cohen, *Understanding Other Minds: Perspectives from Developmental Cognitive Neuroscience,* Oxford: Oxford University Press, 2000, pp. 3–20.

most autistic people have emotions. Examples of emotions are anger, joy, fear, anxiety, love and sadness. They manifest them clearly but often inappropriately—often more clearly than most of us normal people do. Autistic people as a rule do not hide their emotions; unlike us, they are not hypocrites.

The way in which they experience their emotions, however, is probably somewhat different from how we do. When we talk about emotions, we often make reference, metaphorically, to physical sensations: for "sadness" we say pain; we talk about "joy" as being tickled pink; "mourning" makes us feel empty inside; "angst" feels like a knot in our stomach.

I believe that many autistic people experience emotions less metaphorically. For them, angst isn't like feeling a knot in their stomach; angst *is* a knot in their stomach. Joy isn't like being tickled pink—joy *is* an actual tickling sensation.

Sentiments are not the same things as emotions. Examples of sentiments are jealousy, shame, pride, empathy, pity, tenderness, sadism, compassion and friendship. Most autistic people, left to their own means, do not experience sentiments. Simply put, sentiments are affective states that you feel *toward* something, someone or a situation, whereas emotions are affective states you feel *because of* something or someone. I am happy because it's a beautiful day, but I am not happy toward the beautiful day. I feel shame toward the milkman; I shouldn't

Imposters

have complained about the spoiled milk. Sentiments are distinguished from emotions by their intellectual component; they are linked to the understanding of a given social situation, as opposed to the visceral nature of the emotions. You can be happy alone, but you can't be generous or compassionate or empathic all by yourself. This is why sentiments are rarer than emotions in autistic people. Having emotions does not make one a social being. Having sentiments does.

Whether or not the autistic, left to their own devices, can read our emotions or not, one thing is certain—we can transmit our emotions to them if we take the time to try.

I was amazed to learn, some years ago, that many people who work with the autistic do not take the trouble to look them straight in the eye. Looking them straight in the eye is the most important thing we can do. We must load our own eyes with so much warmth, curiosity, fascination and openness—without content or judgment—that no autistic person will be able to resist it. We must spend hours doing this, years, honing that look in our eyes. We must be able to conjure it up at will for each and every eventuality, for each and every autistic person. Our eyes must build a house for them, made-to-order, the door wide open, painted their favorite color, furnished to their taste. We must never stop renewing it, always adding another flourish. Because we can never know when the house is finished, it's up to

them to tell us, with the look in their eyes sent straight
back to us.

During his time of psychological crisis, Martin found
himself standing on the edge of an abyss somewhere between the autistic state wherein one is truly self-sufficient,
thanks to the panoply of self-satisfying activities that autistic people are heir to, and the socialized state, wherein
one relies on interpersonal relationships to give life meaning. As a therapist I had to make a decision: to let him
stay on the autistic, self-sufficient side of the abyss (why
not?—it's very efficient to be self-sufficient; it works) or
take the risk of tempting him to come to the other,
having-feelings-for-other-people side, knowing that he
might fall into the abyss along the way.

I chose right. Martin is becoming generous. He makes
bracelets out of beads and gives them to us as presents,
and he consoles us when we're down; the other day he
walked across the dining room to two very upset *educa-
trices spécialisées*—something about paid vacations—
and gave them a hug. Martin is starting to be proud
when he does something good, and ashamed when he
does something bad. He's acquiring poise: how he holds
his head, the sincerity on his face, the real smile, the real
tears, the tiny signs that tell us that the MartinWho-
ComesAfter is not far away.

*   *   *

I've always been a Tarzan fan. I discovered him when I was ten—an old movie on TV. Nobody'd ever told me about him before. When the movie ended, I was stricken with enormous sorrow. I realized that I'd never see him again. I cried my eyes out. It wasn't until the next day that I saw the notice in the TV listings: the film was the first in a weekly Tarzan series that was going to last six months.

I saw them all. But little by little as the series went by, I felt sadder and sadder. I was in mourning. I realized that one day the series would come to an end, and that I would never see Tarzan again. My parents tried to tell me that there would always be Tarzan movies on TV, that all kids loved Tarzan, and that the networks had a vested interest in putting them on.

Yet my mourning would not cease. It was only gradually that I came to understand the nature of it. I was growing up. One day I would no longer be a child, and I knew that on that day I would stop loving Tarzan. Worse, I knew that the less I loved Tarzan, the more I wouldn't care that I loved him less, since I loved him less.

Every night when I said my prayers, I asked God to not let me stop loving Tarzan. I was afraid. Afraid of losing the HowardWhoCameBefore.

On odd-numbered days when I'm alone, I imagine the MartinWhoComesAfter. I imagine him sitting in front of me. We talk. The discussion is the kind of discussion I've always dreamed of: we talk about a certain subject as one does, and we digress as one does, except that the digressions are not at all the same as one does, nor is the subject the same kind of subject. The voice salad, the free association, the brilliant apples-and-oranges of it all: the World According to Martin.

And then there's this: from time to time, walking down the street, I am intercepted by a curve. The curve is invisible. I can't see it, but I know it's there; it crosses in front of me, there on the sidewalk. It's always the same curve (I could draw it for you if you like). It represents nothing, but for some reason it gives me a feeling of well-being, a sort of consolation. I never talk about it to anyone, but I'm going to bring it up to Martin tomorrow, to see what he says. I'll be anxious to hear his opinion—the unimaginable current opinion of the MartinWhoComesJustBefore the MartinWhoComesAfter.

5

PLAYING THE THERAPEUTIC CHARACTER

Ginette P. smiles all the time. As soon as she hears the doorbell ring, she goes running, happy happy, to welcome you into the institution. Her welcome is always warm. You're surprised to see someone so charming in a psychiatric clinic. She gives you a big smile. She kisses your hand. She joyously escorts you into the building, wherein she attentively takes your wrap . . . whether you want her to or not. You don't want her to, as it turns out, but Ginette insists, still smiling—the same smile as before, the exact same smile as before, which has not budged from her face—and she will take your wrap, this coat here, pulling on it, wrenching it from your back. You lose your balance, almost fall. Totally confused, you start pulling in the opposite direction, slipping and sliding on the small puddle of something chocolate that someone must have spilled here during lunch. Suddenly Ginette lets go of your coat and you go spinning out of control, backward, colliding with the administrative director, who happens to be walking past just now. The two of you effectuate an awkward waltz (or is that a polka? I can never tell), which, it turns out, is propitious, since the administrative director is the person with whom you have an appointment—the New Budget Restrictions—and we all know how awkward it is to break the ice. The two of you stop dancing and head for the stairway. Ginette P. follows you, hysterical with laughter. The administrative director instructs her to go back downstairs, but Ginette doesn't seem to care; she follows you. Things start heating up. Suddenly the doorbell rings again. Ginette stops in her tracks and races back downstairs. She opens the door. She is happy happy. Here we go again. Here we go again.

In the beginning we were all delighted to know Ginette, the never-changing smile ("At least we have one customer who doesn't seem to suffer . . ."), but in short order she started getting on our nerves ("Why does she smile like that all the time? Nobody smiles like that all the time!"). Ginette P. smiles like that all the time, her file tells us, because she is psychotic.

I disagree.

Ginette has two separate handicaps: a mental one and

a diagnostic one. She is mentally retarded, and has a very effective way of getting on people's nerves. She should have been diagnosed with PDD (Pervasive Developmental Disorder), which would have allowed her to be admitted to an integrated kindergarten along with normal children, and later to a school that accepts such youngsters and knows how to educate them. Her condition is congenital; she was born this way. Though her language is extremely limited, she seems to understand much of what we say. Ginette occasionally pretends to beat her head against the wall, imitating others here in an institution where she doesn't really belong. In France, normal-looking retarded people who really, really get on people's nerves are often considered to be psychotic.

There is nothing autistic about Ginette P. Unlike the autistic, Ginette bends over backward to solicit relationships with others. In her it's a symptom (neurotic symbiosis; I'll explain later). This young woman of nineteen years has all the makings of a Lovely and Charming Hostess with the Mostest, except that the Mostest she is with isn't Charming, and on the Lovely front she is equally challenged—her weight is way over, her face a predicament. She picks her nose; she makes herself regurgitate. Her smile (always the same, always the same!) never takes a vacation. This state of affairs in no way stops Ginette from racing to the door every time the buzzer sounds, taking all visitors into her arms, speaking to them in a tiny, whiny voice as enervating as it is incomprehensible.

(It took months to decipher her words: *Go in car, Mommy, Kiss Helen, Art Room.*) Her stocky little silhouette files in and out, in your face every time you turn around, getting in everybody's way ("You again?"); and the big kiss—the BIG, BIG kiss she insists on giving you whether you want it or not, followed by a little tiny pinch that really, really hurts; and voilà, there goes Mademoiselle Ginette, Prom Queen alone in a Promless Land.

Ginette P. does not belong in our clinic, but it's too late now, and at nineteen she is at the age when she must leave us anyway. All French clinical institutions have mile-long waiting lists, and no special school takes adults. We are looking for a local live-in situation for Ginette, but no one has room. Last fall a wonderful residential facility in Belgium, two hours away by car, informed us that they would be happy to take Ginette. The parents categorically refused—no child of theirs was going to go live in Belgium—a notorious pedophile murderer had recently been captured and sent to prison there. (I remind them that Bluebeard was French; they don't care.)

In the interest of establishing a complete educational-therapeutic program tailored to the specific needs of each individual customer—solve what's gone wrong with them, embellish what's gone right—our institution offers some forty-four activities and individual sessions during the course of the week. These include everything from classroom time to African dance, from music and sculpture to psychomotor exercises; psychotherapy sessions (my work with Martin, for example), horseback riding, swimming, hydrotherapy, relaxation (no mean trick), storytelling, language acquisition (PECS and Tallal)*, sensory integration, theater, video (taping themselves, then viewing themselves), library (only 10 percent of our young champions can read, but hey), building maintenance, cooking, gardening, singing (they hum a few bars; we fake it), personal hygiene, beauty shop (in-house), circus skills (in-house), laundry, clay, sculpture, painting, papier-mâché, collage, obstacle course and "culture swapping" (weekly visits to various ethnic-group organizations). In addition to these, we also organize several group trips a year—to the seaside, a horse farm, skiing in the Alps; and individual *séjours thérapeutiques*—week-long or two-week-long sojourns in various specialized living facilities outside of Paris.

It was while driving back from a *séjour thérapeutique* with Ginette that I got to see another side of her. We'd stopped for lunch at a cafeteria on the *autoroute*. Sitting across the table from her, I observed my special partner

---

* PECS: Picture Exchange Communication System, which uses pictograms as a means of exchange that, as words become associated with them, encourages speech. Paula Tallal, a neurolinguist, has created talking CD-ROMs that stretch consonant sounds; studies suggest that some young autistic brains cannot process consonants, because they go by too quickly.

observing the others. Her face was relaxed as she looked over my shoulder at the different people. Suddenly there was no trace of the famous frozen smile. I stared, rapt, as her features melted and molted, participating at a distance in their discussions: two college men, full of enthusiasm, laughing out loud, and Ginette smiling, cocking her head and bouncing in her seat; a middle-aged couple having an argument, and Ginette's forehead furrowing, tears forming in her eyes; a pair of young lovers, staring into each other's eyes . . . they kiss, and Ginette's heart takes wing, as she sits there in front of me with empathy to burn. Now her eyes lower, pan left, settle on my own . . . and bang: here's Mister Smile, back again, covering her face like a gladiator's shield, blocking everything out, keeping everything in. Somewhere a curtain falls, another rises, and off goes Ginette P., whining and posing and kissing and pinching. . . .

At home Ginette persecutes her mother, her mother most of all. A reading of the records indicates that Mrs. P. has a history of mental illness in her family, that she was thus reluctant to have a child, terrified that the trend might continue. Supported by her husband, though, she found the courage to go ahead and get pregnant.

Tough luck.

A colleague and I decide to see Mr. and Mrs. P. once a month, together with Ginette. The sessions are tortuous. The parents take turns reciting litanies of Ginettian obnoxiousness. The list never changes, recounted by both Mom and Dad with a wisp of a smile which is always the same. We want to understand the depths of their psychological disarray. We want to dig deeper, to uncover and analyze the mechanisms at play in this circular system of love, dependence, regret and remorse, and the unbearable double bind these poor people have been living through every day for nearly twenty years. But no. The only useful information we manage to extract from these interminable sessions is what we witness ourselves: in the two years that we've been seeing each other, neither parent has had anything nice to say about their daughter.

Transactional analysis is a form of psychotherapy that has enjoyed great success since the early 1970s. Based on a simplified version of Freud's structural theory of the psyche—the ego, the id and the superego—transactional analysis has been shown to be efficient in the treatment of neurosis. (Neurosis: a dysfunctional but not life-threatening psychological state resulting in behaviors that tend to cause unhappiness, anger, fear, angst or frustration in the subject as well as in the people around him or her.) It postulates certain types of interpersonal relationships, or transactions, that have been conceived to aid us in understanding our ways of interacting with others—family members, coworkers, friends. When these interpersonal relationships—transactions—are dysfunctional, Gestalt techniques are often used to help correct and resolve them. Among these are role-playing, two-chair exercises and regression therapies, often employed in a group setting.

Relationships are analyzed in terms of three ego states: Child, Parent and Adult. In any interpersonal transaction, the participants will unconsciously place themselves in one of these three ego states, according to their individual neurotic tendencies and according to the ego states unconsciously "chosen" by the other people involved in the transaction. Certain people will tend to place themselves in a Child ego state whenever confronted with someone who tends to place himself or herself in the Parent ego state, and vice versa. One person might also unconsciously encourage the other person to assume the Parent position in order to facilitate his or her own natural tendency to assume the Child ego state.

Ego states have subcategories too: Critical Child and Nurturing Child, Critical Parent and Nurturing Parent. The healthiest transactions between grown-ups take place when both participants are in the Adult ego state.

The relationships between Ginette P. and many members of the staff have become as twisted as those that exist between Ginette and her parents. Our institutional role as professional caregivers—that of Nurturing Parent—is constantly being subverted by Ginette, who, by alternating between Nurturing Child (opening the door for us, carrying our bags, kissing us) and Critical Child (pinching us and laughing at us) is forever making us into Critical Parents.

All our staff psychologists believe that Ginette is severely mentally ill (I'll stop saying psychotic now); they talk about her in terms of the "false self," a psychoanalytic construct that is used as an alternative to the term *disassociation* when describing schizophrenia. (Schizophrenia smacks of the asylum, whereas "false self" sounds more like something you'd see on an analyst's divan.) Disassociation is the phenomenon of feeling cut off from your own life experience, of watching yourself go through the motions—it's the "split personality" part of schizophrenia that we often hear about but that many people wrongly confuse with "multiple personality." (The latter occurs when several different people take turns living in one person's head—the "Three Faces of Eve" syndrome.) So much time is spent talking about severe mental illness in our institution that it took years for me to realize that Ginette is just an intellectually deficient individual with an inferiority complex: "I don't deserve to belong to any club that would have me as a member, and I'm going to prove it to you." It probably stems from the message she's been receiving from her parents since the day they realized that their worst nightmare had come true in the person of a mentally ill daughter. Had they been told the truth—that Ginette was retarded rather than insane—things might have turned out differently.

Neuroses are serious, but are not usually referred to as a mental illness (as in "My daughter is mentally ill"). Still, Ginette P. makes me think of what we call "borderline" psychoses—conditions that walk the fine line between neurosis and psychosis. Borderline patients are extremely difficult to deal with. Their particular psychopathology causes them to pretend to be even more pathological than they truly are. They are traditionally not quite insane enough to be considered mentally incompetent—incapable of living on their own in society—yet their pathology keeps their psychologists and psychiatrists perpetually off balance, never knowing exactly how to respond, how to reason with someone who is not quite reasonable yet who is not unreasonable enough to not reason with.

Borderline people are often known for their brilliance and cleverness; they have a way of talking circles around you—usually about themselves and what, as their therapist, you're doing wrong. That this state of psychopathological affairs should show up in someone as unlikely as Ginette P. is tantamount to a scoop.

Like a borderline person, the mentally retarded Ginette plays at being mentally retarded. She deliberately screws up simple tasks of which she is capable, even though it would be almost normal for her to screw them up anyway. She occasionally takes to beating her head against the wall, and though it is obvious to everyone that she is doing this to attract attention, it is not uncommon for severely mentally retarded people to beat their heads against the wall (when frustrated, for example).

ˋ Although neuroses like those of Ginette are successfully treatable by techniques such as transactional analysis, her language and comprehension deficits (no one knows for sure how much of what we say she really understands) compromise any therapeutic care plan we can manage to come up with. Mentally handicapped and very neurotic Ginette plays the role of a mentally handicapped neurotic. Her unconscious, appropriately neurotic goal is to realize the message that her parents have been sending her from the day she was born: *You are not lovable.*

(*Note:* Guilt is inevitable in all parents of all handicapped children, and its effects are always insidious. It makes the whole family neurotic; no one is spared. The goal of our family counseling sessions is to help everyone see things more clearly, find ways for all of them to get along more easily in the life they've been saddled with or born into. These sessions usually fail because we are unfortunately not insightful or clever enough to get the job done right.)

The fluctuating and paradoxical roles that Ginette constantly plays cut deep into the weaknesses of our staff. Her different pathologies—something for everyone—get us where we live. In becoming neurotic about her, we have become incapable of overcoming the momentum of her own neurotic motors, and thus incapable of treating her neurosis. She has managed to run circles around us, making us do her dirty work by refusing her membership in the one club that *has* to have her for a member: the people who are paid to care for her.

A population of severely affected autistic-spectrum individuals (and the occasional possibly borderline ones) requires certain exceptional efforts on the part of the people who work with them. We must be prepared to start from scratch every day, to perpetually reinvent our invented methods. Our energy must be as gigantic as our results are infinitesimal, because these results—should there actually be any—are so slow to come that we might not even recognize them when they arrive. Whatever progress our work might enact in the people with whom we work—the capacity to relate, the capacity to share, the capacity to empathize, the capacity to be patient—will be directly proportional to our own individual human qualities. Our tools are ourselves. If we don't possess these qualities, our customers never will.

Operating on the hypothesis that Ginette's neurotic, annoying behavior stems from the message she's received from her family for so many years, our mission ought to be to find a way to undo the message, replace it with a counter-message. This counter-message must be clear, straightforward and simple enough to avoid any ambiguity that would allow the neurotic mechanisms to subvert it. It must be delivered in such a way that Ginette cannot help but receive it and integrate it into her already defensive psyche. The protocol must be institutionally cogent, airtight. We have no time to lose.

I conceive a plan: from this day on, every time we cross Ginette's path, we will take a moment to engage her—stop her in her tracks if necessary. We will look her straight in the eye, and, using all the forms of communication that human beings possess (tone of voice, facial expression, body language, vocabulary), we will let her know that we see her as a young woman who is capable, personable, genuine, intelligent, generous, clear and well-meaning. A different Ginette, a Ginette we imagine as being possible—an image of herself that we will systematically send her every time we cross her path. It will be by means of this image—this composite of our individual images of this young woman, rich in their differences, strong in their likenesses—that Ginette will eventually be able to reconstruct herself psychologically, in the same way that every human being structures himself or herself from the day they are born: through the image of themselves that they receive from the people around them.

What do we wish for Ginette P.? As annoying as her behavior may be, it is only in imagining what we wish for her that we will be able to see what needs to be done, and how best to go about doing it. Criticizing her for her "hypocrisy" will only feed the hypocrisy we wish to starve. It is her principal defense mechanism, operating on everyone around her, psychologically designed to prove that she is, as she's always been led to believe, unlovable. We could perhaps discuss this very mechanism with her, as would a normal psychotherapist with a normally neurotic client. But Ginette's neurosis is seated in real and severe mental retardation—she understands simple commands ("Go get the dishes in the kitchen and set the table"; "Take the mail up to the office"), but she herself possesses a vocabulary of barely ten words, most of which are incomprehensibly pronounced (her parents translated them for us when she was admitted). This state of affairs is complicated by the fact that she constantly playacts being more retarded than she is. Were we to discuss her neurosis with her, we could never be sure of how much she truly understood. (Not to mention the fact that she is so widely unloved by the staff that the tone of voice employed by them during such discussions would tend to have the same negative effect as outright criticism.) No, the only sure way to address this young woman in a believably positive way is to imagine her otherwise, not as a gorgeous cover girl or as a brilliant intellectual but as the capable, convivial, sensitive, honest person (borderline or neurotic or retarded or not) that she very well could become should we do our job well enough.

To do our job well enough in this case means, first and foremost, to find the necessary human resources within ourselves to render us equal to the task. Being equal to the task in this case means being capable of rigorously applying the necessary therapeutic protocol. The necessary protocol at hand involves imagining another possible Ginette, and relating to her as such.

But with every passing day, the staff becomes ever more impatient with her. Imagining another, different Ginette turns out to be too much to ask of them. They say they're sorry, but they can't do it. They say they can't do it and that they're not sorry. Some criticize the protocol, contending not only that it is impossible to put into effect but that in the end it's detrimental to the well-being of the client: responding to Ginette's hypocrisy with our own hypocrisy will only make things worse. We just don't like her. It's our God-given right.

Ginette will soon leave our clinic. She has not changed. We have failed her. That she isn't autistic is not the reason. We simply couldn't get past our own natural reactions, our personal taste in human beings. We were not willing enough to act as if we believed.

The relative success or failure of our work depends greatly on the personal relationship that we are, or are not, able to establish with our patients. This relationship is a tool—a human tool, customized and conceived expressly for the task at hand. Moreover, as difficult as the task at hand may be, the fashioning of this necessary tool may be more difficult still. This is because its very existence depends on the capacities of both people concerned—caregiver and client alike. This tool is sometimes referred to as the therapeutic alliance.

It is difficult to establish a therapeutic alliance with most autistic people, because their abilities to relate to others are by definition restricted.

How to proceed?

With the autistic the first step, though easier said than done, is clear: we must figure out how to attract their attention. To attract their attention, we must be interesting in their eyes. To be interesting in their eyes, we must often invent a special way of being, a specific personality. This personality will differ according to the person we are addressing. It must be made-to-order, customized in detail and reinvented daily for each individual with whom we come into therapeutic contact, tailored to their desires as well as to their needs; according to their taste. In this situation, the customer is always right.

To make ourselves interesting to a particular autistic person, we must first understand what exactly he or she finds interesting. Since the therapeutic alliance is by definition based on mutual respect for the individuality of all concerned—client and therapist alike—it is necessary, at least at first, to accord the autistic their particular "autisms." This may be done by simply leaving them alone. The better way, of course, is to participate. As a general rule, participating demonstrates empathy, acceptance and even admiration. Where autism is concerned, especially nonverbal autism, demonstrating is more efficient than explaining. The clearest form of demonstrated empathy is imitation.

All caregivers are not created equal when it comes to the art of imitation. Some innate talent is required. Any small well-meaning attempt, though, is worthy. As mentioned in a previous chapter, invested imitation of the autistic may give one a decent idea of what it feels like to be them. In many, albeit subtle, ways this experience feeds our therapeutic instincts, sharpens our clinical intuition. Faced with an explosive or critical situation concerning an autistic individual—panic, suffering, anger or sorrow—the ability to imagine, "If I were that person, what would make me feel better right now?" is priceless.

Accepting the autisms of the autistic—being able to appreciate them, even—demands certain human sensibilities that are not given to everyone. When one finds oneself face-to-face with an autistic person—someone who is completely closed off from the environment, who won't look at you, who doesn't seem to hear you, who is violent with you, who screams and spits at you, who seems more like a living rag doll than a living person—it is normal to feel reticent. We are afraid to invade their space. We are afraid to upset them. We are afraid to not honor their choice of solitude. We wonder what distance to keep, what time to take, what signals to watch for, what signs to obey. At first we stay and watch and wait, doing nothing else, often for hours and hours, all the while making sure—through our geographical position in the room (I usually stay about ten feet away at first, at a forty-five-degree angle, thus allowing the person to look at me or not look at me with equal ease); through our body language (open, passive); through our observably relaxed state (attained, no matter how stressed we really are, by conscious breathing and muscular release); through our facial expression (neutral yet interested)—that we are thoroughly available to him or her. Like the fox in *The Little Prince,* the autistic person will let us know "when . . ." and "to what extent. . . ."

The comings and goings of daily life provide us with a multitude of opportunities to make ourselves interesting to these unusual people. Though gift shopping for the autistic at Bloomingdale's can be problematical, offering them a cookie here and there, a stick of chewing gum or a Coke, is not. (I prefer stick chewing gum to the Chiclet-tablet style—you can roll it up in front of them, roll it lengthwise, unroll it, roll it halfway, jiggle it around. . . .) Despite the normal rules and regulations that all healthy institutions and homes must maintain (when and where one may be allowed to have a snack, chew gum or blow a bubble) and most conventional wisdom concerning the benefits of rigorous constancy for the autistic person (always putting the same things in the same places, never altering the sequence of events), sneaking someone the occasional Snickers for no particular reason can often be a useful brick in the building of a therapeutic alliance.

If, as Freud contended, dreams are the "royal road to the unconscious," then the royal road to the autistic psyche is its sensoriality: touch, sound, smell, sight and proprioception. It is principally through these "roads" that we may hope to establish affective relationships with these incredibly special people: merit their interest, earn their confidence.

Once this is done, we may move on to pre-therapeutic exercises. . . .

For example, the Terrifying Curse of the Limp Hands. The professional prerequisite for this treatment modality is knowing how to transform oneself into Frankenstein's Monster: hold your arms straight out in front of you, your hands dangling limply from the wrists, dishraglike; then drool (optional) while moaning in a cadaverous voice, "*The Terrifying Curse of the Limp Hands . . . the Terrifying Curse of the Limp Hands. . . .*" Now stalk the patient all over the clinic or school until you have him or her cornered—preferably in front of onlookers, who will be the next victims—and, after ceremoniously dangling the said limp hands in front of his or her face, smush them around in it and issue a bloodcurdling scream (optional).

161

Remembering one's roots is important. One may wish to pay tribute to the old-fashioned psychiatric traditions of yesteryear by bringing them back—the sedative injection, for example. One begins by announcing to the patient (regardless of whether he or she understands—it's the tone that counts) that this injection is inevitable and will be very, very painful. Thus warned, the patient will watch as the county mental health worker withdraws the hypodermic needle (which strangely resembles a ballpoint pen) from his pocket. The county mental health worker then produces the vial (which strangely resembles a ballpoint pen cap) of chlorpromazine and shakes it vigorously. The hypodermic needle is inserted into the vial and the tube fills with invisible chlorpromazine as the mental health worker, holding the vial/cap and the pen/hypodermic in one hand, draws the index finger and thumb of the other hand down the sides of the hypodermic/pen, filling it. Holding the pen/hypodermic up to the light, he taps the cylinder to make sure there are no air bubbles, pushes the point into the patient's arm and, screaming (well, someone has to scream), pushes his thumb back up the hypodermic/pen, injecting the heinous drug. He then pulls out the pen, rubs the spot and stops screaming. He informs the patient that he or she will soon feel better, and asks what he or she would say to some chocolate milk.

Some like to be tattooed (drawn on . . . washable ink,

please). Others may be better off tickled. Still others may appreciate weird mouth sounds against their ears, or the occasional burp.

To help Martin be kinder to his mother at home (less cloying and obsessional), I screw the idea of being kind into his head. It goes in halfway up the left side, in the middle. (The idea of not-being-afraid-of-becoming-an-adult, however, gets screwed in in the back, just under the cowlick.)

Every morning Damien insists that I sing "The Star-Spangled Banner" with high-fives in tempo. This is followed by my honking his nose, which is followed by my turning his ears into shortwave radio knobs which, when turned this way and that, emit the appropriate whiny-whistling frequency sounds (hum and whistle at the same time, cool). Then I have to place each of my hands four inches away from each of his ears, which he gets clapped by himself, swaying his head from side to side. This accomplished, he makes me unscrew his cranium and lift it off with a popping noise (optional), out of which I must withdraw his pulsating brain (mime). This routine, which ends by my cracking an imaginary egg on Damien's head and letting the insides flow down the sides of his face, must never vary in order.

Dirka backs up toward me. It's Tchaikovsky time again. Standing behind her, I take her two elbows into my hands, and together we conduct the London Symphony

Orchestra in the Tchaikovsky Violin Concerto in D (second movement: andante, hummed by guess who). As always, the crescendo finishes with Dirka in ecstasy.

Benoit A., usually inert, is dragging me up the stairs. Though it isn't Monday, he wants his massage. Every Monday a Rolfing specialist comes to the clinic to give Benoit his deep massage therapy. Rolfing, invented in Germany by Ida Rolf for her own handicapped daughter, is a technique whereby one systematically separates the musculature from the skeleton, thereby allowing all the muscles, which have grown twisted and stuck from daily life, to "fall" naturally into place again, thus enabling the person to regain the postural-gravitational equilibrium he or she was born with. For this technique to succeed, it is necessary to dig very deeply, and some people find the experience excruciatingly painful. Benoit A. never stops laughing.

Virginie B. runs across the room to shake my hand for the fifth time today. Virginie is pathologically shy, and shaking people's hands means a great deal to her. She usually just waves from afar. Certain staff members decline to shake Virginie's hand more than once a day. They believe that a single daily handshake is sufficient in society and that Virginie should be made to understand this. Virginie does not understand this. There are many things that Virginie does not understand about society. That is why she is in our institution. Shaking people's hands means a great deal to her. I will shake Virginie's hand as often as she is willing to shake mine, and I will never, ever miss an opportunity to wave at her from afar.

When Abdelkader K. explodes—results: tables overturned, furniture smashed, wrists (his own) bitten into bloody pulps—he may sometimes be calmed down by a simple glass of water. It is important that the water be either very hot or very cold. The sensation of an abrupt internal temperature change shocks him out of his terror and back into our world.

The daily physical dealings with a clientele such as ours may demand a certain level of fitness on the part of the staff. I sometimes find it incumbent on myself, during or in the aftermath of a self-injurious tantrum, to carry a full-grown adult male in my arms or on my back. This relatively extravagant act allows me to communicate without any possible ambiguity two important things to the person in question: (1) I am stronger than you are; and (2) No matter how tough the going gets, you can always count on me.

All these are examples of how to attract and keep the attention of people whose attention is notoriously difficult to attract. This attraction, obligatorily mutual (otherwise we wouldn't take the trouble), is the foundation upon which other varied personal relations may be founded, all of which are prerequisites to trust. This trust, which is subject to perpetual maintenance, is what we are referring to when we talk about the therapeutic alliance. Though I would never go so far as to say that once these relationships are established anything is possible, I say that without them very little will be.

The ability to find within ourselves a particular way of being with the autistic, and the ability to put it into action on request, demand certain natural gifts that are not always present in special education teachers and clinical psychologists: imagination, intuition, inventiveness, playfulness. And yet these ways of being are, I believe, indispensable to the successful accompaniment, education and therapeutic care of the population with whom we have chosen to work. They are our *therapeutic characters.*

Playing a therapeutic character is not a matter of "becoming someone else" or "hiding behind a mask." It is a matter of calling up certain parts of our own true personalities—parts that we might not call upon often—and putting them to work in the service of someone else, in the same simple way that normal parents find it in themselves to "play the meanie" in the service of disciplining their child.

This act is neither more nor less "hypocritical" than that of the actor who plays Romeo on the stage and who must for the length of the scene convince himself that he is madly in love with the actress playing Juliet. If the actor does his job well, his resulting psychological state will not be one of pretending—it will be one of authentically loving the Juliet he imagines, the Juliet he invents for the occasion and projects onto the actress standing before him, a Juliet who is necessarily lovable because she has been custom-made to be so in the imagination of the actor. Under the current circumstances, imagining a lovable Juliet and loving her for the prescribed amount of time is as much a part of his obligatory professional mandate as is putting on his makeup and memorizing his lines.

Imagining is a professional skill as necessary for those working in our profession as it is for actors. We must be able to imagine in advance the reasonable progress that our young clients are capable of making, if we are to be efficient in planning their educational and therapeutic activities. To be able to conceive of how to get them from here to there, it is necessary to know what "there" looks like.

One cannot imagine something that one knows nothing of. It is always necessary to have some kind of information, empirically observed by ourselves or by someone else, which we process through our own thoughts and feelings. (Even a biochemist must, in some measure, think and have feelings about the microorganisms under his or her microscope.) Imagining is the affective psychological processing of a situation outside ourselves that does not exist. I can imagine my brother who may be a hundred miles away—see him clearly in my mind's eye—but what I imagine will never exactly correspond to the empirical reality of my brother at that moment. Imagining is thus necessarily empathic in nature and therefore of great importance, both in the constitution of an appropriate care plan and in the constitution of a therapeutic alliance.

But how are we to empathize with someone who is very, very different from ourselves? In many ways profoundly autistic people are not like us at all. They do not manifest the same behaviors; they do not manifest the same emotional responses. To assume out of hand that they "have emotions like you and me" is not necessarily doing them a favor. Yes, they have the same emotions as we do: joy, sorrow, angst, fear; but the nature of their emotions, the ways in which they are experienced (viscerally, intellectually) and the ways in which they are generated—what it is that makes the autistic person joyful, angst-ridden, fearful—are often likely to be beyond our ken. For us to feel what they are feeling becomes something of a feat.

In daily life, empathy is something that happens by itself. We listen to our next-door neighbors talk about the recent death of their dog and we automatically empathize by calling up similar situations that we ourselves have lived through. But since we are not autistic and never have been, the ability to feel what our clients are feeling— be they classically autistic or otherwise extraordinary— is a talent that must be developed through practice. We must use our own projections and identifications, as efficient or inefficient as they may be, to imagine what it feels like to be Ginette, Damien or Martin, in their minds and in their bodies.

Until we can feel what it's like to be them, we will never be able to imagine how it would feel to be them as they change, as they evolve, as they become otherwise. Until we can imagine what they feel as they change, we will never be able to find in ourselves the particular way to facilitate their journey along the way.

It is this "way of being"—our therapeutic character, born of empathy and played for real—that will supply, in part, the necessary and specific human environment within which these incredible people will be able to re-create themselves.

This world was not meant for the autistic. Here upon our huge little earth there are myriad thousands of cultures, each with its own language, looks, folkways, mores, music, art, habits and laws; so original, so rich, that we are proud. How is it, then, that we rejoice in all our different peoples, but not in our different people?

On even-numbered days I tell myself that if that's the way it's going to be, fine; I'll just go and buy a desert island, and I'll collect everyone on the face of the earth who's autistic and we'll sail away to it, far from these societies of so-called *Homo sapiens*—these societies that were made for so many kinds of human beings except them—and together, we'll live like people.

On odd-numbered days I tell myself the opposite.

What exactly is suffering made of? Ours? Theirs? What exactly is the difference between the two? How much does it weigh? What is the opposite of suffering made of? What a surprise if in the end it turned out to be made of sharing, teaching, discovering, opening our eyes, broadening our horizons? What if in the end the opposite of suffering was simply learning what it's like to be each other?

ACKNOWLEDGMENT

I thank Ann Harris, who never let me let myself off the hook.

ABOUT THE AUTHOR

HOWARD BUTEN, Ph.D., is the founder of the Adam Shelton Center in Paris, and divides his time between Paris and New York. He also practices two other professions: as a performing artist in Europe, he is the theatrical clown-mime Buffo, and he is the author of seven novels published in France. His first novel, *Burt,* was also published in the United States in 1981, and was republished here in 2000 as *When I Was Five I Killed Myself.*